Work-based Learning in Clinical Settings

Insights from socio-cultural perspectives

Edited by

VIV COOK
Senior Lecturer in Medical Education
Barts and the London School of Medicine and Dentistry
Queen Mary, University of London

CAROLINE DALY
Reader
Institute of Education, University of London

and

MARK NEWMAN
Reader
Assistant Director, Health and Wellbeing
Institute of Education, University of London

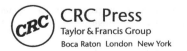

CRC Press
Taylor & Francis Group
Boca Raton London New York

CRC Press is an imprint of the
Taylor & Francis Group, an **informa** business

T0321412

CRC Press
Taylor & Francis Group
6000 Broken Sound Parkway NW, Suite 300
Boca Raton, FL 33487-2742

© 2012 by Viv Cook, Caroline Daly and Mark Newman
CRC Press is an imprint of Taylor & Francis Group, an Informa business

No claim to original U.S. Government works

Printed on acid-free paper
Version Date: 20161202

International Standard Book Number-13: 978-1-84619-495-5 (Paperback)

Visit the Taylor & Francis Web site at
http://www.taylorandfrancis.com

and the CRC Press Web site at
http://www.crcpress.com

Contents

Contents

About the editors

Viv Cook (v.cook@qmul.ac.uk) is a Senior Lecturer in Medical Education at Barts and the London School of Medicine and Dentistry, Queen Mary, University of London. She was seconded for 2 years to the Centre for Excellence in Work-based Learning for Education Professionals at the Institute of Education, University of London, completing a funded project on the workplace learning of novice clinical teachers. She led the development of the Researching Learning for Clinical Practice network, which aimed to support colleagues completing postgraduate qualifications in education. She is a faculty developer, training and advising medical educators to enhance the learning of medical students and trainees at postgraduate level.

Caroline Daly (c.daly@ioe.ac.uk) is Reader at the Institute of Education, University of London, where for 3 years she was Assistant Director of the Centre for Excellence in Work-based Learning for Education Professionals. She was a founder member of the Researching Learning for Clinical Practice network, and works with colleagues in medical education to support cross-sector networking and dissemination of research into professional education. Her research background is in professional learning, e-learning and teacher education. She has published widely for both research and practitioner audiences, and recently co-authored *Key Issues in e-Learning Research and Practice* (Continuum, 2011).

Mark Newman (m.newman@ioe.ac.uk) is Reader at the Institute of Education, University of London, where he is Assistant Director: Health and Wellbeing. He is Assistant Director of the Evidence for Policy and Practice Information and Coordinating Centre (EPPI-Centre) and Programme Leader for the MA in Clinical Education. He was a founder member of the Researching Learning for Clinical Practice network, and works with colleagues in clinical education to support cross-sector networking and dissemination of research into professional education. His research interests include the design of effective learning environments in clinical education and the use of research evidence to inform policy and practice decision-making.

Contributors

Jeff Bezemer (j.bezemer@ioe.ac.uk) is a Senior Research Fellow at the Institute of Education, University of London, and Deputy Director of MODE, a node of the National Centre for Research Methods. He is interested in ethnography, learning and communication.

Alan Bleakley (alan.bleakley@pms.ac.uk) is Professor of Medical Education and Deputy Director of the Institute of Clinical Education at Peninsula Medical School, Universities of Exeter and Plymouth. He has an interest in socio-cultural aspects of learning and aesthetics of medical education.

Alexandra Cope (Alexandra.cope07@imperial.ac.uk) is a Clinical Research Fellow at Imperial College London and a Specialist Registrar in General Surgery in the Oxford Deanery. She is interested in postgraduate surgical education.

Tim Dornan (t.dornan@maastrichtuniversity.nl) is Professor of Medical Education at Maastricht University, the Netherlands. From a background in internal medicine and endocrinology, he completed a masters degree in health professions education in 2002 and a PhD on the topic of clinical workplace learning in 2006, both at Maastricht University. He now works solely as an education researcher. He headed Manchester's medical education research group until his move to Maastricht in 2009. His interests include clinical workplace learning, socio-cultural theory, qualitative research and bibliographic methodology.

Karen Evans (k.evans@ioe.ac.uk) is Professor and Chair in Education (Lifelong Learning) at the Institute of Education, University of London. Her main fields of research are learning in life and work transitions, and learning in and through the workplace. She is a leading researcher in the UK Economic and Social Research Council Centre for Learning and Life Chances in Knowledge Economies and

Societies. She has directed major studies of work and learning in Britain and internationally, in collaboration with a wide range of education professionals and 'professionals who educate'. Her books include *The Sage Handbook of Workplace Learning* (2011); *Improving Literacy at Work* (2011); *Learning, Work and Social Responsibility* (2009); *Improving Workplace Learning* (2006); *Reconnection: Countering Social Exclusion through Situated Learning* (2004); *Working to Learn* (2002); and *Learning and Work in the Risk Society* (2000). She is an Academician of the Academy of Social Sciences.

Will Gibson (w.gibson@ioe.ac.uk) is a Senior Lecturer in Social Research Methodology at the Institute of Education, University of London. He is interested in interactional sociology and the empirical exploration of technologically mediated social activities.

Mary Gobbi (mog1@soton.ac.uk) is a Senior Lecturer in Nursing at the Faculty of Health Sciences, University of Southampton. Mary is an ethnographer and educational evaluator with a critical care nursing background. Her academic and research interests include the learning and development of clinical competence through simulation and daily healthcare practice.

Vikram Jha (Vikram.Jha@Liverpool.ac.uk) is Professor of Medical Education and Head of Undergraduate Medical School, University of Liverpool. His research interest is in professionalism, workplace learning and patient involvement in medical education.

Roger Kneebone (r.kneebone@imperial.ac.uk) is Professor of Surgical Education at Imperial College London. His research is focused on simulation and the contextualisation of clinical learning. He has developed innovative approaches to learning and assessing clinical procedures, using hybrid combinations of models and simulated patients.

Gunther Kress (g.kress@ioe.ac.uk) is Professor of Semiotics and Education and Director of the Centre for Multimodal Research at the Institute of Education, University of London. He is interested in questions of meaning and its semiotic realisations in interrelation with social and cultural organisation.

Dirk vom Lehn (dirk.vom_lehn@kcl.ac.uk) is Lecturer in Marketing at King's College London. His research is largely concerned with social interaction and technology in optometric practices and in museums and galleries.

Clare Morris (Clare.Morris@beds.ac.uk) is Associate Dean, Postgraduate Medical School, University of Bedfordshire. Her research interests include work-based learning and faculty development in medicine and dentistry.

Stephen O'Connor (stephen.oconnor@beds.ac.uk) is Reader in the Internationalisation of Health Professions' Education at the University of Bedfordshire. Interests include the development of quality standards for doctoral education and international curricula for cancer nurses in Europe. He is also a steering committee member and teaches on the European Union-funded programme 'Leadership for Public Health in Europe'.

Trudie Roberts (t.roberts@leeds.ac.uk) is the Professor of Medical Education and Director of the Leeds Institute of Medical Education at the University of Leeds. Her interests include the areas around assessing competence and performance, professionalism and developing expertise in medicine.

Zeryab Setna (zeryabsetna@yahoo.com) is a Consultant Obstetrician and Gynaecologist at the Lady Dufferin Hospital, Karachi, Pakistan. His research interest is in workplace learning and assessment.

Helena Webb (Helena.webb@kcl.ac.uk) is a research associate in the Department of Management at King's College London. She uses ethnomethodology and conversation analysis to conduct video-based studies of healthcare practices. She has been involved in studies of obesity clinics as well as optometry practices.

Copyrights
Material reproduced with kind permission from Informa Healthcare and Elsevier.

Introduction
Working to learn in clinical practice

Karen Evans

LEARNING IN AND THROUGH PRACTICE LIES AT THE HEART OF clinician education. Advances in clinical knowledge and transformations in the contexts of clinical practice have made visible the complexities and challenges of this learning. These advances have rendered the wider professional education of which it forms a part increasingly provisional. In tandem, the search for deeper understandings of what it actually means to learn and to teach in clinical settings has intensified. Work-based learning (WBL) is a field recently come of age and now maturing as it elaborates its distinctive conceptual and theoretical lenses through collaborative relationships with researchers in a range of professions. The Researching Learning for Clinical Practice Group had its origins in the WLE Centre (Centre for Excellence in Work-based Learning for Education Professionals), which I was privileged to co-direct between 2004 and 2009. In this context, the Researching Learning for Clinical Practice Group has been one of the most enterprising and critically engaged groups with which I have had the privilege to work. The group brought together educational researchers, academics and practitioners from a wide range of clinical and mainstream education institutions that share an interest in the learning of practitioners in workplace settings. It grew to include a wide group of approximately 150 medical education practitioners in undergraduate and postgraduate contexts, working with professionals involved in diagnosis, therapy, prevention, health promotion, rehabilitation and/or management of care. These include medical doctors, nurses, midwives, physiotherapists, speech therapists, health visitors and radiographers. This book is one product of the rich interactions generated in and through that network, a response to the growing demand from regulators, educators, clinicians and students for conceptual and methodological tools that can help to develop learning in professional healthcare contexts. Setting the scene in this introduction is both an honour and a challenge.

WBL is sometimes regarded as a problematic and uncomfortable term associated with old-fashioned notions of apprenticeship or occupations that have technical requirements but which cannot properly be regarded as 'professional'. Yet the significance of the workplace as a site for learning and becoming a professional has long been recognised in the 'first generation' professions of architecture, engineering and medicine, at all stages of the education and professional development process. This volume fundamentally reframes thinking about clinical practice as WBL in the health and medical professions, drawing creatively on intellectual tools and theoretical positions associated with socio-cultural perspectives.

WBL is, at root, about relationships between the fundamental human, social processes of working and learning. It is best understood as learning that derives its purposes for the contexts of work. Theories and perspectives cluster in ways that are of particular significance to an inclusive understanding of learning in, for and through practice. Important clusters focus respectively on cognition and expertise, and on practice-based, organisational learning. Critical theories bring alternative insights that attend to power relations in ways that challenge some dominant assumptions. Other clusters focus on questions of identity and social life or knowledge management. In an authoritative review of the field, Sawchuk (2011) has concluded that each of these domains contains robust lines of inquiry: empirically grounded; theoretically informed; encompassing a sufficient, if not complete, set of factors and considerations; and offering challenges to a 'mechanistic view of reality' (p.167). The field, having defined itself as a set of competing perspectives, is now ready for a more dialogic approach in which robust lines of inquiry are opened up more fully to an exploration of overlaps, gaps and points of connection. This volume contributes to that process. We need to understand better the diversity of purposes that derive from the contexts of practice, the scope and nature of clinical practice and how different forms of knowledge can be put to work in the development of pedagogic and curriculum strategies. We also, I argue, need to think in social-ecological terms about the relationships between work and learning as they play out through the dynamics of different scales of activity: societal, organisational and personal. While the agency of the learning individual is often foregrounded as highly significant for learning in and through clinical practice, this learning is essentially relationships oriented, collaborative rather than a solo activity, and has to be understood in its political, regulatory and institutional contexts. The contributions in this volume begin a debate on the different lenses that can be employed within a broadly socio-cultural frame of reference. A dialogic approach challenges us to consider, as we read: are there combinations of lenses that are sufficiently complementary to sharpen our understandings of these complex matters, while sharing underlying assumptions?

Exploring tensions

There is a marked divergence between the university-appropriated conceptions of WBL that takes place in practice placements and the concepts associated with 'workplace learning'. For 'workplace' perspectives that emphasise the social, cultural and political dynamics of workplaces (in companies, hospitals, schools or third sector organisations), the lenses used bring into focus the work practices that other lenses sometimes miss. However, these lenses can also produce 'tunnel visions' of a different kind. They distance themselves from versions of WBL conceived of as a class of higher education programmes, since such conceptions often disconnect the use of work as a resource for learning from the political realities and social relations of the workplace as experienced by employees. For those whose priorities are rooted in workplace learning, the 'work experience' or the 'placement' is seen as a source of learning that involves only a partial workplace presence, which excludes many of the features of the employer–employee relationships that are so crucial in influencing workplace learning experiences.

The use of socio-cultural lenses does reveal how learning at work is embedded in production processes and social relations. However, situated analyses of work and learning also often fail to make connections between the organised and planned (often termed 'formal') types of programmes that incorporate elements of WBL and the workplace learning that is embedded in 'everyday work' within the social dynamics of organisations – between the workplace and wider work–life relationships and the careers of practitioners as they move into and out of communities of social practice (and, indeed, participate in several simultaneously). When the analytic lenses of the social organisation of learning are used exclusively in the 'here and now' of workplace activity, the biographical learning and pathways of the learning individual are often out of focus or beyond the range of view.

Can approaches that use theoretical concepts for analysing the constitution of practice connect with those that focus on the challenges, problems and opportunities that arise for people in their particular professional and learning trajectories? To what extent can practice be used as a resource to rethink theory and how can better understandings of power relations in the workplace make visible the assumptions that underpin public policy in this field? This volume potentially offers some ways of navigating these tensions, through methodological innovation in researching the complexities of learning in and through clinical practice.

Making new connections

One research cluster, recently burgeoning in its influence, focuses on micro-interaction in workplace activities. This domain is strongly represented in the present volume, which provides detailed insights into naturally occurring processes in everyday clinical workplace interactions. The preoccupation with organisational factors that is often apparent in other research domains can cause us to lose sight of the complexities of practice and how social practices both reflect and shape culture and social structures, including work organisations. Theoretical perspectives linked to strong lines of research inquiry developed by Lave (2009) and by Luff *et al.* (2000) have been used in fine-grained analyses of what occurs in practice and how it occurs. Micro-interaction studies rooted in the theoretical traditions of socio-linguistics and semiotics have used forms of discourse and conversation analysis to shed light on how practice is reproduced, renewed and innovated. Chapter 7, by Jeff Bezemer and his colleagues, takes this theoretical tradition into the operating theatre, to explore what the language we use to talk about learning actually means. This work connects with constructs of situated learning in its focus on social interaction and physical activity. Learning is embedded in a cultural–social context of everyday activities. Learning always takes place in relation to people and their contexts, and in communities of social practice. While Lave (2009), whose concepts have been appropriated, critiqued and misrepresented in various ways, has in 2009 revisited her accounts to explain their theoretical roots in historical materialism, the concept of the community of practice – in which learning is constituted through the sharing of purposeful activity – continues to be explored for its explanatory value in the fields of professional learning in ways that are both illustrated and problematised in the chapters by Viv Cook (Chapter 2), Will Gibson *et al.* (Chapter 9) and Clare Morris (Chapters 1 and 5). Meanwhile actor-network theory disrupts dominant discourses in ways that are expertly illustrated by Alan Bleakley in Chapter 8.

Research clusters overlap in ways that have already produced some key points of connection. At the intersections between micro-interaction/communication research and cognition/expertise studies such as those of Eraut (2007, 2004, 2000), studies such as Gheradi's (Gheradi, 2000; Gherardi and Nicolini, 2006) have shown how the 'texture' of work organisations is continuously created and recreated through the interplay of historical, cultural, material, structural and normative factors. It can thus connect creatively with research on 'ways of knowing', 'knowing in practice' and the range of knowledge forms (procedural, declarative, tacit, implicit, reactive) present in practice. Practice-based studies are often criticised for neglecting power relations, particularly those that have adopted uncritical perspectives on the workings of communities of practice. At the intersection of these 'situated' theories of practice and critical theories of power relations in workplace learning, Engeström's work (Engeström, 2008, 2001; Engeström and Kerosuo, 2007) has drawn attention to the workplace dynamics of power and control through detailed, practice-focused analyses of organisational change processes. These approaches differ from interaction studies and analyses of situated cognition in their focus on boundary crossings and multiple meditations between 'subject' and 'object' within divisions of labour, community and workplace rules, as Clare Morris's Chapter 5 explains.

Research that focuses on the immediate work setting or group has to be situated in an understanding of the dynamics of wider institutional and regulatory contexts. Although there are strengths in understanding learning as participation, this approach often fails to recognise that, in paid work, the employment relationship is often contradictory and sometimes antagonistic in ways that fundamentally influence participation and learning. Activity theory attempts to link local working practices with wider organisational frameworks, but sometimes it takes the wider regulatory frameworks that underpin the relationship between managers and workers for granted, paying relatively little attention to individuals. For the purposes of this volume, keeping different scales of activity in view is essential for an understanding of practice in clinical settings. Learning in and through practice has to be explored at different scales of activity, 'zooming' in and out (to use a metaphor derived from the use of an Internet map or viewing tool) to gain an integrated view of the 'whole' and how the integral parts come together in ways that are best understood interdependently and holistically, in cultural context.

From the starting point that workplaces are crucially important sites for learning, the contributions in this volume show how analytical perspectives on WBL can be used to explore the social and organisational mediation of learning in clinical practice, with the aim of making sense of what it is to teach and learn in different clinical settings. Such sense-making is inextricably linked with questions of what triggered the learning in the first place. According to whether the learner is a trainee, registrar, new general practitioner, a new entrant to work or an experienced doctor with supervisory responsibilities, learning takes place very differently, depending on the specific setting, on the status and role of the learner and on his or her prior work and learning experience. There are aspects of WBL that are specific to the profession. Each sector has its own history of policy and qualification development, its own culture of skills and practice recognition and improvement. WBL activities such as projects, cases or problem-solving can take their impetus from the job, from the wider environment of work or from changes in the knowledge base. They might start with a work challenge that has to be solved, such as the need to overcome a technical or procedural problem, or they might be triggered by the need to share knowledge and experience with others as part of participatory management strategies. Finding ways of responding to unforeseen occurrences or new circumstances can engage teams in intra-organisational and inter-professional learning, while professional networks often respond to challenges by forms of co-operation that operate far beyond organisational boundaries.

Rethinking purposes and perspectives

So learning in and through clinical practice takes place individually and collectively in the workplace as well as beyond its physical boundaries, and the purposes of an expanded WBL derive from the highly differentiated contexts of work, employment and professional practice that people experience. The purposes that derive from the contexts of work are wider ranging than often assumed (*see* Table I.1).

Each of these purposes can be understood from the perspectives of practitioner and professional body interests as well as those of the employer, and from the perspectives of, for example, user reference groups of patients and families, the pursuit of National Health Service reform agendas, and the interests of the wider society. For example, the adoption of 'brands' and mission statements has made corporate enculturation processes more visible; 'on the job' enculturation of clinical practitioners may be compliant or resistant. Practice improvement is a purpose that is often driven from the 'bottom up' in organisations; innovation is more often 'top down'. Increasingly, practitioner-driven innovation (see Evans and Waite, 2010) is a focus of attention, with implications for knowledge flows and power relations between levels of the workforce. In the development of wider capabilities, the impetus may come from the organisation or the profession as well as the professionals' individual interests in positioning themselves for career development. In ethics, equity and social justice, theorising practice as a way of resolving professional concerns (see Guile and Young, 1995) can lead to the development and improvement of models and procedures. The organisation of learning through trades union structures and professional representative bodies foregrounds social justice, recognising that workplace cultures can foster, for example, the learning of racism or gender stereotyping (see Evans *et al.*, 2006; Allan *et al.*, 2004) as readily as the learning of tolerance and co-operation.

TABLE I.1 The purposes derived from work contexts

Purpose	Relates to ...
Enculturation	The processes of 'learning how we do things here'
Competence, licence to practise	The learning necessary for performance to occupational and professional standards, demands of increasing regulation, health and safety standards, keeping abreast of new systems and technologies
Improving practice, innovation and renewal	Learning to do what has not been done before; this involves significant WBL and occurs every time a new set of demands is introduced, particularly in the public sector
Wider capabilities	The development of professional and occupational capabilities; learning to 'do the next job' as well as the current one; learning to work in different cultures and environments
Equity, ethics and social justice	The processes of systematically reflecting on practice within a set of professional concerns about ethics, values, priorities and procedures
Vocational/ professional identity development	New entrants 'thinking and feeling' their way into a vocation or profession and coming to identify with it and with others who participate in it; experienced workers developing and reconstructing identities in and through work as positions, roles and contexts change

The dynamics of knowledge and pedagogy have always to be kept in view in this expanded view of learning in and through clinical practice. The pursuit of all these purposes brings the fundamentally different logics of different types of knowledge (personal, procedural, ethical, propositional, tacit, embodied) into play. At the heart of WBL lie processes of knowledge recontextualisation, as knowledge is put to work in different environments. Questions of knowledge and how context mediates knowledge permeate this volume. All knowledge, I argue, has a context in which it was originally generated. Contexts are often thought of as settings or places, but contexts extend to the 'schools of thought', the traditions and norms of practice, the life experiences in which knowledge of different kinds is generated. For knowledge generated and practised in one context to be put to work in new and different contexts, it has to be recontextualised in ways that simultaneously engage with and change those practices, traditions and experiences. The theory–practice challenge, as I have argued elsewhere (Evans *et al.*, 2010) is to uncover how chains of recontextualisation can be forged iteratively to support learning. This approach has extended beyond Bernstein's position that concepts change as they move from their disciplinary origins and become a part of a curriculum (Barnett, 2006; Bernstein, 2000), to draw on van Oers's (1998) cultural-historical idea that concepts are an integral part of practice and change as practice varies from one sector or workplace to another. Both of these notions can be substantially expanded through socio-cultural understandings of the ways in which practitioners themselves change as they work with concepts and practices and the extent to which this process may spur innovation in workplaces as well as educational contexts. Stephen O'Connor, in Chapter 4, has developed Bernstein's theories in a different, but related way to generate insights into nursing pedagogic practice. Mary Gobbi (Chapter 6) explores the significance of forms of knowledge that are tacit and embodied, while Vikram Jha *et al.* (Chapter 3) focus on the challenges of developing assessment in guided learning. Multiple forms of knowledge are in play where teaching involves guiding clinicians at the limits of what they know and where unpredictability is inherent in the context.

A social-ecological metaphor provides a way into understanding the complexity of factors that impact directly or indirectly on clinical workplace learning without losing sight of the dynamics of the whole. Every contextual factor and every person contributing or influenced is part of a complex ecology, or system of social relations and relationships that sustains the system through a set of interdependencies. According to Weaver-Hightower's (2008) overview, the four categories – actors, relationships, environments and structures, and processes – lie at the heart of social-ecological analyses. These differ in the degree of significance accorded to personal agency, through which actors 'depending on their resources and power, are able to change ecological systems for their own benefit' (p.156). Because ecologies are self-sustaining through interdependencies that operate without centralised controls, individuals and groups have spaces in which to exercise agency in ways that can influence the whole dynamic, through the interdependencies involved – agency is exercised through bounded spaces rather than structured deterministically. These perspectives are significant for the ways in which practitioners can use the workplace as a learning space for ends that extend far beyond it.

A key hypothesis, explored in Chapter 10, by Caroline Daly, is that WBL can be enhanced through the use of creative technologies. Drawing in new intellectual resources to deepen and expand our understanding and practice is made more possible, more feasible with the digital technologies now available. 'Mobility' in learning itself has new meanings as the locations and social spaces in which work is carried out diversify and work itself becomes mobile and distributed. When learning in and through clinical practice is understood as part of a wider dynamic, the analysis has to include the recognition that workers both are part of the work system and have lives outside it; they are engaged in multiple overlapping structures and social practices. Well-being ultimately depends on the interplay of personal and professional roles and interests. A social ecology of learning strives to understand interrelationships between motivations and capacities to act in the world, the cultural practices of everyday living and working and the social and technological structures of the worlds we inhabit.

This book encourages practitioners to embrace conceptual diversity and contextual variation. Contributors explain their understandings of the ways in which contexts mediate learning, through structures, networks, relationships, activities and artefacts. The scope is multi-professional and multi-specialty, covering nursing, ophthalmology, and medical and surgical practice communities. Furthermore the chapters are rooted in different social science traditions – philosophical, psychological, sociological – offering a range of epistemological and methodological approaches as well as intellectual tools for rethinking specific teaching and learning practices. The editors have, herein, created a new and challenging learning space for those ready to think in new ways about learning in clinical practice. Prepare to be stimulated and challenged.

References

Allan, H. T., Larsen, J. A., Bryan, K., *et al.* (2004) The social reproduction of institutional racism: internationally recruited nurses' experiences of the British health services. *Diversity in Health and Social Care*, 1(2), 117–26.

Barnett, M. (2006) Vocational knowledge and vocational pedagogy. In: M. Young and J. Gamble (eds) *Knowledge, Curriculum and Qualifications for South African Further Education*. Cape Town, HSRC Press, pp.143–57.

Bernstein, B. (2000) *Pedagogy, Symbolic Control and Identity: theory, research critique*. Rev. edn. Lanham, MD, Rowman & Littlefield Publishers.

Engeström, Y. (2001) Expansive learning at work: toward an activity theoretical reconceptualization. *Journal of Education and Work*, 14(1), 133–56.

Engeström, Y. (2008) Enriching activity theory without shortcuts. *Interacting with Computers*, 20(2), 256–9.

Engeström, Y. and Kerosuo, H. (2007) From workplace learning to inter-organizational learning and back: the contribution of activity theory. *Journal of Workplace Learning*, 19(6), 336–42.

Eraut, M. (2000) Non-formal learning and tacit knowledge in professional work. *British Journal of Educational Psychology*, 70(1), 113–36.

Eraut, M. (2004) Informal learning in the workplace. *Studies in Continuing Education*, 26(2), 247–74.

Eraut, M. (2007) Learning from other people in the workplace. *Oxford Review of Education*, 33(4), 403–22.

Evans, K., Hodkinson, P., Rainbird, H., *et al.* (2006) *Improving Workplace Learning*. Abingdon, Routledge.

Evans, K., Guile, D., Harris, J., *et al.* (2010) Putting knowledge to work: a new approach. *Nurse Education Today*, 30(3), 245–51.

Evans, K., Guile, D. and Harris, J. (2011) Rethinking work-based learning for education professionals and professionals who educate. In: M. Malloch, L. Cairns, K. Evans, *et al.* (eds) *The Sage Handbook of Workplace Learning*. London, Sage, pp.149–62.

Evans, K. and Waite, E. (2010) Stimulating the innovation potential of routine workers through workplace learning. *TRANSFER: European Review of Labour and Research*, 16(2), 243–58.

Gherardi, D. (2000) Practice-based theorizing on learning and knowing in organizations. *Organization*, 7(2), 211–23.

Gherardi, D. and Nicolini, D. (2006) *Organizational Knowledge: the texture of workplace learning*. London, Blackwell.

Guile, D. and Young, M. (1995) Further professional development and FE teachers: setting a new agenda for work-based learning. In: I. Woodward (ed.) *Continuing Professional Development Issues in Design and Delivery*. London, Cassell, pp.235–68.

Lave, J. (2009) *Apprenticeship in Critical Ethnographic Practice*. Chicago, IL, University of Chicago Press.

Luff, P., Hindmarsh, J. and Heath, C. (eds) (2000) *Workplace Studies: recovering work practice and informing system design*. New York, NY, Cambridge University Press.

Sawchuk, P. (2011) Researching workplace learning: an overview and critique. In: M. Malloch, L. Cairns, K. Evans, *et al.* (eds) *The Sage Handbook of Workplace Learning*. London, Sage, pp.165–80.

Van Oers, B. (1998) The fallacy of decontextualisation. *Mind, Culture, and Activity*, 5(2), 143–52.

Weaver-Hightower, M. B. (2008) An ecology metaphor for educational policy analysis: a call to complexity. *Educational Researcher*, 37(3), 153–6.

1

Reimagining 'the firm'

Clinical attachments as time spent in communities of practice

Clare Morris

THE WORKPLACE HAS LONG BEEN A SIGNIFICANT SITE FOR MEDICAL learning at all stages of education and training. Calls for 'early patient contact' (GMC, 1993) have led to a gradual demise of the traditional preclinical–clinical divide in undergraduate years, with students spending time in clinical workplaces from year one. Despite the significant investment of resource in undergraduate 'attachments' of this nature, there are increasing concerns about new graduates' preparedness for professional practice and the lack of opportunities for 'hands on' work before graduation (Illing *et al.*, 2008). Indeed, the relaunch of *Tomorrow's Doctors* (GMC, 2009) has been accompanied with calls to reinstate the traditions of old, arguing that clinical attachments, shadowing and new 'student assistantships' should have greater prominence (GMC, 2009). These calls arise alongside concerns about the demise of medical apprenticeship (Dornan, 2005), the loss of the clinical 'firm', the impact of UK National Health Service reform on medical training and a shift toward competency-based models in postgraduate years (Tooke, 2007). There has perhaps never been a better time to research workplace-based learning in medicine; the challenge is perhaps to identify the types of conceptual and theoretical tools that best enable us to do this.

In this chapter, I explore the use of Lave and Wenger's conceptions of *communities of practice* and *legitimate peripheral participation* as potentially useful analytical tools that offer new insights into medical students' experiences of learning in the workplace (Wenger, 1998; Lave and Wenger, 1991). In particular,

I explore the extent to which students 'clinical attachments' can be reconceptualised as times spent in communities of practice. In order to do this I start with an exploration of Lave and Wenger's work, concluding with a distillation of what I see as the core underpinning tenets. This leads me to consider the ways in which these core tenets might be 'operationalised' to guide a socio-cultural research inquiry into medical student learning. The value of this approach is illustrated by a research study that investigated how clinical teachers support undergraduate learning in medical workplaces (Morris, 2009).

'Rescuing the idea of apprenticeship'

The term 'communities of practice' is often evoked in learning literature and is gradually creeping into descriptions of medical learning and practice (PMETB, 2008). To trace its origins, it is necessary to turn to the seminal work of Jean Lave, a social anthropologist, and Etienne Wenger, a teacher and educational researcher, who set out 'to rescue the idea of apprenticeship' 2 decades ago (Lave and Wenger, 1991, p.29). They noted that while the term 'apprenticeship' was in regular use, its meaning was unclear and it was often used synonymously (and unhelpfully) with the term 'situated learning'. Their analysis arises from a series of studies of apprenticeship, spanning Yucatec midwives, Vai and Gola tailors, naval quartermasters, meat cutters and non-drinking alcoholics. Their thesis, in essence, is that learning is an 'integral and inseparable aspect of social practice', characterised as 'Legitimate Peripheral Participation in Communities of Practice' (Lave and Wenger, 1991, p.31).

There is merit in emphasising the shifts in thinking necessary in order to fully appreciate the merit of their work, which has been argued to transform the 'assumptions and metaphors guiding the study of learning' (Hughes *et al.*, 2007). Sfard (1998), in particular, contrasts the 'dominant' metaphor for learning (learning-as-acquisition) with the metaphor emerging from their work, that of learning-as-participation. She argues that while the perceived goal of learning-as-acquisition is the ever-greater accumulation of knowledge and skills, the goal of learning-as-participation is to become a fully participant member of a community. If the learning-as-participation metaphor is applied to the purposes and outcomes of medical students' clinical attachments, less emphasis might be given to the acquisition of clinical knowledge or skills, and more to facilitating student participation in the medical practices of the (disciplinary) communities they join.

Sfard (1998) argues that the choice of metaphor is highly consequential with regard to the pedagogic strategies employed and the approaches to educational research and scholarship adopted. For example, the learning-as-acquisition metaphor may privilege certain types of learning experiences (e.g. lectures and clinical skills sessions) or certain types of assessments (e.g. multiple-choice questions and objective structured clinical examinations) in pursuit of this goal. In contrast, the learning-as-participation metaphor might privilege participative learning experiences (e.g. clinical attachments, shadowing, student apprentice-ships) or assessment methods (e.g. workplace-based assessments or multi-source feedback). It is worth noting that Sfard (1998) cautions against the adoption of a single metaphor, a point picked up by Bleakley (2006), who argues in favour of the productive tension of these competing ideas, suggesting a need to choose those with the most explanatory power for the issues being explored.

Arnseth (2008), a key analyst in the field of socio-cultural research, argues that Lave and Wenger's major contribution is that

> they make use of this notion of practice in order to construe a reformulation of thinking and learning. Thus, they treat thinking and learning as something that is constituted in the lived-in-world – the world as it is experienced in social practice. (p.294)

This idea, that learning is an integral, inseparable part of social practice, leads us to think differently about medical thinking and learning in the workplace. When a healthcare team gather around a patient's bed to review patient management, or a surgical team almost wordlessly move through the unchoreographed yet seamless operation, learning is happening as part of shared 'social' practice, whether made explicit or otherwise. Lave and Wenger (1991) offer up this analytic viewpoint by inviting us to draw upon two linked concepts: 'legitimate peripheral participation' and 'communities of practice'. Taken as a conceptual 'whole' (they caution against deconstruction), legitimate peripheral participation becomes, in their words, 'a descriptor of engagement in social practice that entails learning as an integral constituent' (p.35).

Legitimate peripheral participation focuses attention on the ways in which 'newcomers' to a community (e.g. medical students or trainees) are invited into the community and are engaged (or otherwise) in increasingly meaningful activity that enables them to become full participants in the practices of that community. This view on learning moves us beyond understandings of learning that focus on abilities to take part in new activities or perform new tasks. As Lave and

Wenger (1991) note, these activities only have meaning in relation to broader systems of relations. For example, a student's ability to perform venepuncture is given meaning when the sample of blood they take from the consenting patient is analysed by the pathologist and the findings discussed in the wider context of a team managing that patient's care. By being involved in discussions of patient care, the student learns not only 'from talk' but also 'to talk', being socialised into ways of thinking about and talking about patients. By inviting the student to take the blood sample, his or her practice becomes integral to the shared practice of the patient care team. Over time therefore, the student comes to *belong* to that community and to *become* a doctor through such processes. This view of learning therefore invites us to consider issues of professional identity formation. In other words, to look at the ways in which medical students are invited to take part, indeed to 'be a part' of the work of that community and, in so doing, start to 'become' a doctor.

The communities of practice concept is introduced in Lave and Wenger's (1991) joint text, but is (as they would acknowledge) only loosely defined at this point. They argue that the term 'community', in this sense, is both 'crucial and subtle', indicating not only the shared technical knowledge and skills of community members but also the relations between community members and the activities they engage in and the world. Communities are delineated in their text on the basis of the so-called 'reproduction cycles' from newcomer to old-timer, as new members become full participants. In later work, Wenger (1998) offers a three-dimensional distinction, focused on 'mutual engagement, joint enterprise and a shared repertoire' (p.73). He also cautions against using the term synonymously with teams, groups or networks. This underdevelopment of the communities of practice concept poses some difficulties in using this idea analytically in research, particularly in relation to delineating an appropriate unit of analysis for research. It is difficult to research a community of practice if it is not clear where it begins and ends.

A full exploration or critique of the concept is beyond the scope of this chapter, and can be found elsewhere (e.g. see Hughes *et al.*, 2007) and so only the key concepts, or 'core tenets', are given here: first, the view that learning is an integral part of social practice; second, that communities of practice can be identified and defined by common expertise and shared practices; third, learning has a central defining process, that of legitimate peripheral participation, a process enabling the development of the expertise necessary to enable access and full participation in a community; fourth, learning involves the *construction of identities* (processes of belonging and becoming); and, finally, it is recognised that language is a central part of practice, not in terms of learning from talk, but rather in terms of *learning to talk* – a process of talking one's way into the expertise (Wenger, 1998; Lave and Wenger, 1991). In the rest of this chapter, the aim is to explore how these core tenets can be put to use as analytical tools to research medical learning.

Rethinking medical apprenticeship

Some commentators have been critical of the strongly individualised 'cognitive' conceptions of learning that appear to dominate the medical education literatures and the atheoretical nature of much medical education research (Teunissen, 2010; Norman, 2007). Bleakley (2006) and Swanwick (2005), in particular, identify the desirability of broadening the ways in which learning is conceptualised in medical education and the importance of drawing upon appropriate conceptual tools to do this. More recently, Mann (2011) has argued that socio-cultural learning theories offer the medical profession new ways to think about themselves and their practices.

In my own research work, I have drawn on Lave and Wenger's conceptions to help me rethink medical apprenticeship. This rethinking has been part of a wider study seeking to make explicit the ways in which clinical teachers support medical student learning in the workplace. My starting premise was that Lave and Wenger's (1991) work offered new ways into exploring learning and working relationships, practices and tools.

Their work also led me to ask different types of questions about medical student learning in the workplace. Specifically, if learning can be characterised as 'legitimate peripheral participation in communities of practice', to what extent can medical students' attachments be viewed as time spent in communities of practice? Furthermore, how might the analytical lens of 'legitimate peripheral participation' help make sense of the learning that happens (or otherwise) on clinical attachments?

Researching medical student learning on attachments

A key concern I had when designing my research, was finding the most appropriate unit of analysis and aligned research methods. Säljö describes this as a scholarly creation, allowing researchers to put theoretical perspectives to use

(Säljö, 2009, 2007). This is not a straightforward process. Matusov (2007), for example, notes that while most socio-cultural researchers would argue that the individual is not an appropriate unit of analysis, they differ in their positions on what is. If learning is seen as part of social practice, embedded in the everyday practices of a community, the chosen unit of analysis should seek to embrace and explore such complexities. Lave was a social anthropologist immersed in ethnographic studies of naturally occurring apprenticeship; tracing a full 'transformational cycle' from newcomer to old-timer may be possible in such circumstances. However, these methods do not readily translate to practitioner research seeking to make sense of medical student learning. Most researchers are constrained by resource issues and what is feasible in terms of access to the field. Therefore, in designing my research study, a decision was made to focus on the experiences of medical students, across all years of their course, recognising that this would potentially afford insights into a wide range of 'communities' and might offer some insights into the complexities of learning in clinical workplaces. At the time this research was started (in 2004), there was limited debate or exploration of research methods congruent with a socio-cultural enquiry (beyond the ethnographic work alluded to). A bespoke methodological approach was therefore developed, the goal being to make explicit the ways in which Lave and Wenger's (1991) ideas about learning were being put to use in the design and implementation of the study. Three key methods were used: literature review and reframing, observation of medical student learning in the workplace, and interviews. Examples of these ways of working follow.

Literature review and reframing

A first step in many studies will be a review of the literature. Given the lack of research on undergraduate medical education arising from a socio-cultural tradition, there was no immediately congruent literature base on which to draw. However, there is a large literature exploring student and trainee experiences of learning in the workplace that emanates from other different theoretical traditions, but which shares similar concerns. These studies explore issues of context, of practice and of 'cultural' issues.

To illustrate, it is possible to take the previously articulated 'core tenets' arising from Lave and Wenger's (1991) work to look anew at studies published in key medical education journals in recent years. Studies exploring the types of learning that emerge during ward rounds of different types (e.g. Kuper *et al.*,

2010; Walton and Steinert, 2010) or in particular disciplines (e.g. Baler *et al.*, 2010) could be seen as studies that are exploring the idea of learning being part of social practice. The emphasis given to learning in different settings (e.g. community versus hospital-based attachments) or learning within certain specialty settings (e.g. surgical versus medical attachments) can be reframed in terms of learning happening within communities of practice. These studies may well signal particular cultural traditions and practices implicitly, even if they are not dealt with explicitly. Studies exploring issues around preparedness for practice or the activity of medical students during clinical attachments can readily be viewed through the analytical lens of legitimate peripheral participation. Again, implicitly, if not explicitly, these studies are exploring the extent to which medical students are enabled to become full participants in medical communities, at or around the time of graduation. Issues of learning involving the construction of identities emerge in the literatures on developing medical professionalism. The idea of language being a central part of practice is explored in work by Lingard *et al.* (2003), and highlighted as important by Swanwick (2005), for example.

In reframing literature in this way, it is possible to argue that while there may be few studies of medical learning and practice that are explicitly located in the socio-cultural traditions, there are many studies of medical education that explore the key issues identified in the socio-cultural tradition. This would support the idea, therefore, that the conceptual tools offered have potential value in researching these fields. The socio-cultural approach also provides a different way of 'reading' the literatures currently available, shedding new light on potential fields of inquiry.

Observation of medical student learning

Ethnographic observational methods have an immediate appeal to researchers interested in the ways in which medical students are invited to engage in the everyday activity of the workplaces they enter on attachment. In my own research, there were two prime considerations to take into account. First, the issue of access and resource; my research was not funded and therefore had to 'fit' into the other demands of professional life. Prolonged periods of observation, however desirable, were not an option. Second, there was a theoretical issue to consider. Classically, ethnographic methods are adopted where there is an intention to reveal the purposes of particular practices or activities (as was the case with Lave and Wenger's original studies). In my study, however, the observed activities were chosen because of their known purposes (to support medical student learning on attachments). My research was therefore more 'framed' than might be the case in a traditional ethnography. I did, however, share common concerns of ethnographers about the status and authenticity of observational data, the methods of observation and data recording employed, the nature of the relationship between the researchers and researched, and the analytic approaches adopted (Atkinson and Hammersley, 1998). These concerns were addressed by seeking a transparency of approach, e.g. by being clear about the nature of relationships, by ensuring ethical practices; by detailing and triangulating methods; and by adopting a reflexive approach that brings researcher concerns to the fore. My research study, in effect, explicitly built in observational 'biases', with the approach being one of selective attention (to doctor–student mediated activity in the workplace) and encoding (viewed through a particular theoretical lens). By making these planned 'biases' explicit, it is possible to argue the value of drawing upon the methodological tools of ethnography in new ways.

In my study, a short period of (non) participant observation was used as a way of exploring the potential analytic value of the conceptual tools identified and to inform the development of interview guides for later discussions with medical students. The term 'participant observation' is being used broadly here; participation is limited by the specific context in which it occurs. I am not medically qualified and therefore it would be highly inappropriate for me to participate by engaging in everyday medical practice. Explicit access to observe medical students within the workplace was granted and opportunities were arranged, across different contexts and years of the undergraduate course. While the amount of time spent observing was relatively brief (seven sessions of 1–3 hours), it is worth noting the biographical resources being brought to the work. As a speech and language therapist, I had spent a decade working in secondary care contexts, working with medical colleagues. Prior to the study, I had also spent a year as a faculty developer working with clinical teachers, both within and away from their workplaces, focusing on clinical teaching practices (including observation of teaching). Although 'an outsider' to the communities observed, I felt I had enough 'inside' experience to have a meaningful understanding of this workplace and had established trusting relationships with the medical colleagues who allowed me to observe them at work with students.

During observed sessions, I was a silent observer (unless invited to comment by a medical teacher), but, where possible, I spoke to the teacher and/or students before or after the observed session in order to get a sense of how exceptional the session had been, to identify the rationale for the approaches used (where known) and to obtain student perceptions of the purpose and usefulness of the session. Following the observations, I wrote up the free notes in the form of a narrative, adding any questions arising or interpretive possibilities. In these periods of writing up, I aimed to explore the extent to which it was possible to conceptualise observed attachments as times spent in communities of practice. In particular, I sought to identify common expertise within the community, evidence of legitimate peripheral participation, and the learning resources embedded in community practice that enabled this. A summary description of each observed community was produced, exploring these strands. The purpose of this chapter is not to present research findings per se. However, excerpts of observational notes illustrate links between observations and the analytic lenses being used.

For example, the following note, seen through the lens of legitimate peripheral participation, illuminates the ways in which the student is drawn into shared practice in a rheumatology outpatient clinic:

> Note: Consultant and student were reviewing the case notes and test results of a patient due to be seen in clinic whose rheumatoid arthritis had been poorly controlled when last seen. The teacher handed the blood test results to the student and asked him to comment on whether the change of medication had helped and why that might be. When the patient arrived the medical student was invited to explain the results of the test to the patient in terms of whether her arthritis was improving.

The next note was made following observations in an antenatal clinic and reveals something of the ways in which students begin to construct their professional identity. The tension between preparations for examinations (in this case an OSCE – objective structured clinical examination) and 'real world' practice also raises questions about the extent to which student practice is aligned to the practices of the communities they join.

> Note: Medical student starts to take the blood pressure of a pregnant patient in the antenatal clinic. The consultant stopped the student to ask if he was doing it 'as if for the OSCE' or the way he would do it if he was the doctor. They agreed the student would do the procedure 'as if for an OSCE' and having done so, the student was then asked to say how he would normally do it in clinic.

A third note reveals something of the idea that students learn 'to talk' as well as learn from talk. During several of the observations, I observed consultants 'coach' students into preferred ways of presenting patients, with implicit structures being made more explicit through these processes.

> Note: The Consultant was interrupted between cases by a trainee who needed guidance with an urgent issue. The trainee commenced with a verbal account of the patient and what had happened – mid account the medical teacher interjected to explain to the observing medical student that the patient's baby was lying in a breech position – at this point the trainee did a dramatic heel of hand on forehead gesture and commented 'Damn! I knew I'd forget it – it was the main thing … I was rehearsing what I was going to say outside the door – I can't believe I did that!'

Interpreting these participative interactions through the analytic lenses provided by communities of practice and legitimate peripheral participation afforded new insights and some provisional conclusions about the nature of medical students' workplace-based learning experiences. These provisional conclusions were then used to shape questions used to guide discussions with medical students, both in one-to-one interviews and in focus groups.

Interviews: talking about learning on attachment

My interviews were theoretically driven. My starting point was that particular conceptual tools (the core tenets identified earlier) could be used to shed light on and make sense of the learning experiences of medical students. A 'topic guide' was developed as a point of reference for the semi-structured interviews with medical students, both one-to-one and in groups. This guide was developed with reference to the core tenets of communities of practice and subsequently focused by the observational study described earlier. In particular, the observational work led me to a closer focus on the ways in which medical students perceive their attachments as times spent in communities of practice (or otherwise). The interview topic guide had questions (and 'probes') designed to explore the ways in which medical students are able to recognise and make explicit specific work-based learning practices and the value they attach to particular practices. In developing the questions, I wished to find ways to explore the opportunities for legitimate peripheral participation created for students and the ways in which medical teachers displayed expertise that was helpful to the development of students' own practices as future doctors.

Interview questions were operationalised in language that would be familiar and understandable to medical students. For example, the following question is one of a number attempting to explore legitimate peripheral participation.

Topic Guide Question 10

I am really interested in the idea that when you are on attachments you become part of a 'firm' – I wonder to what extent you really do become part of the firm or team – a participating member with a part to play?

Probes
- Do you feel part of team?
- What helps you/stops you belonging?
- What is your role – what do you bring to the firm?

Conditions placed on 'access to the field' limited the ways in which I was able to recruit to interviews. Posters seeking volunteers were placed around campus and 10 students responded. Fortunately, they spanned years two to six of the undergraduate degree; between them they had experience of over 30 different clinical attachments. In terms of gender, ethnicity, age and prior educational experiences they were broadly representative of the medical student population. I chose to use both individual (four students) and group (six students) interviews. The former were felt to allow exploration of ideas in depth and offer the opportunity to follow the interview through to a logical conclusion. The group interviews offered a balance to what might be a very personalised, narrow perspective; interaction between participants could potentially shed light on differences of perspective. Interviews lasted between 45 and 75 minutes and were recorded and subsequently transcribed in full. They were then broadly 'content coded' by marking up transcripts on the basis of which research question or questions they offered insights into (as there were four questions in the wider study).

Therefore, in the data analysis stage, rather than seeking emerging themes (a commonly adopted approach when analysing qualitative data), the aim was to use the core tenets of communities of practice to explore medical student attachments in different clinical practice settings or firms. As part of this, I was therefore interested to explore the extent to which medical students identified and made explicit the apparent 'cultural' practices of each of the medical communities they were attached to. I was also interested in finding out whether they felt that they needed to adapt their own ways of acting in order to be accepted within these communities and therefore to access the types of learning activities arising from engaging in the everyday work of these communities. In looking closely at all of the transcripts, I found 18 examples of students talking about their experiences of clinical attachments that were felt to shed light on these issues. A few of these are presented here as exemplars; it is interesting to note that these responses also shed light on the struggles encountered by students as they construct their future identities as doctors.

> It's like in the city, dress the same, carry the same briefcase, try to fit in.

> I think you find yourself changing without knowing it and you look back and think god, I never would have done that a year ago, I never would have behaved that way but you find yourself doing it because it is easier almost to fit in with everyone else.

> It's about behaving the way the patient wants you to behave as a doctor – it's what they expect of a doctor which I find difficult – I don't want to be like that – I don't want to put on a front of being overly confident and knowing exactly.

> The breast surgery firm I loved but ultimately the doctors were surgeons and surgeons, I find, have a certain way of acting and handling themselves which I feel quite intimidating and I don't think I'd fit in terribly well with that – and I did think I would fit in better on a medical firm – ultimately that will be important part of how I choose my career but in the meantime you do want to fit in.

> Half the degree is socialisation to become a doctor and the other half of it is learning the skills you need – and it really is a process of changing – and you have to change – it's almost like you can't become your own person until you've actually done it and become a doctor and then you can do it your own way.

This mapping of responses against research questions and concerns allowed me to test out the utility of the core tenets of communities of practice as a way of developing new understandings about medical student learning in the workplace. The core tenets gave me a language to think about and talk about student learning in new ways. Ultimately, I concluded that clinical attachments could be seen as times spent in communities of practice, at least in a descriptive sense. Students made distinctions between communities of practice at a number of different levels, in relation to the types of learning opportunities afforded and the teaching and learning relations. Observed and described practices are congruent with the idea that learning happens through legitimate peripheral participation. This was visibly apparent in the teaching of clinical and consultation skills, but also suggested in the opportunities given to students to think through and talk through the diagnosis and management of patients, for example. Students in this study appeared sensitive to the 'cultural norms' of different communities, in relation to a range of features including codes of dress, communication, behaviour and practice. These sensitivities appear to enable students to adopt or express appropriate professional identities in order to facilitate access into these communities and thereby increase opportunities for legitimate peripheral participation. It also led students to question career pathways and the 'type' of doctor they wished to become.

However, students varied significantly in the extent to which they both recognised and valued the workplace as a site for learning in their undergraduate years and the extent to which they appeared to seek out and accept opportunities to engage in workplace-based practices. The interplay between their individual 'agency' (in terms of seeking out and engaging with opportunities) and the 'affordances of the workplace' (in inviting them to do so) is complex and an area meriting further exploration, perhaps drawing on some of the conceptual tools offered by Billett (2009). He is critical of what he sees as the down-playing of the individual in the socio-cultural literature, arguing that they

> de-emphasize not only the contributions of the personal in terms of individuals' cognitive experience (i.e. what they know and through which they experience) and the interests and intentions that shape that experience but also the negotiations between the social suggestion and the inherently personal process of knowledge construal and construction. (p.35)

My research study sought to make sense of workplace-based learning experiences and the value of looking at these through a particular theoretical lens, guided by the learning-as-participation metaphor. It is important to remember that these experiences sit within the formal curriculum of undergraduate medicine, making them quite distinct from the types of apprenticeship being studied by Lave and Wenger (1991). The power of the 'learning-as-acquisition' metaphor in shaping students' beliefs about 'good teaching' and 'valuable learning' experiences should not be overlooked.

The workplace continues to be a valued (albeit contested) site for learning in medical education and training. National Health Service reform has placed considerable challenges upon those responsible for supporting this type of learning. The conceptual tools offered by communities of practice and legitimate peripheral participation offer new ways of thinking about, talking about and researching medical learning. In drawing upon these tools, we are better able to make explicit to ourselves and to our learners, the learning value of engaging in everyday activities within the workplace. In turn, this may help us to better prepare new graduates for the challenges they face as they enter the workplace as doctors, not students.

References

Arnseth, H. (2008) Activity theory and situated learning theory: contrasting views of educational practice. *Pedagogy, Culture and Society*, 16(3), 289–302.

Atkinson, P. and Hammersley, M. (1998) Ethnography and participant observation. In: N. Denzin and Y. Lincoln (eds) *Strategies of Qualitative Enquiry*. London, Sage, pp.110–36.

Balmer, D. F., Master, C. L., Richards, B. F., *et al.* (2010) An ethnographic study of attending rounds in general paediatrics, understanding the ritual. *Medical Education*, 44(11), 1105–16.

Billett, S. (2009) Conceptualizing learning experiences: contributions and mediations of the social, personal and brute. *Mind, Culture, and Activity*, 16(1), 32–47.

Bleakley, A. (2006) Broadening conceptions of learning in medical education: the message from teamworking. *Medical Education*, 40(2), 150–7.

Dornan, T. (2005) Osler, Flexner, apprenticeship and 'the new medical education'. *Journal of the Royal Society of Medicine*, 98(3), 91–5.

General Medical Council (GMC) (1993) *Tomorrow's Doctors*. 1st edn. Available from: www.gmc-uk.org/Tomorrows_Doctors_1993.pdf_25397206.pdf (accessed 26 February 2011).

General Medical Council (GMC) (2009) *Tomorrow's Doctors*. 3rd edn. Available from: www.gmc-uk.org/education/undergraduate/tomorrows_doctors_2009.asp (accessed 2 January 2011).

Hughes, J., Jewson, N. and Unwin, L. (eds) (2007) *Communities of Practice: critical perspectives*. London, Routledge.

Illing, J., Morrow, G., Kergon, C *et al.* (2008) *How Prepared are Medical Graduates to Begin Practice? A comparison of three diverse medical schools*. Available from: www.gmc-uk.org/about/research/research_commissioned_1.asp (accessed 2 January 2011).

Kuper, A., Nedden, N. Z., Etchells, E., *et al.* (2010) Teaching and learning in morbidity and mortality rounds: an ethnographic study. *Medical Education*, 44(6), 559–69.

Lave, J. and Wenger, E. (1991) *Situated Learning: legitimate peripheral participation*. Cambridge, Cambridge University Press.

Lingard, L., Schryer, C., Garwood, K., *et al.* (2003) 'Talking the talk': school and workplace genre tension in clerkship case presentations. *Medical Education*, 37(7), 612–20.

Mann, K. (2011) Theoretical perspectives in medical education: past experience and future possibilities. *Medical Education*, 45(1), 60–68.

Matusov, E. (2007) In search of 'the appropriate' unit of analysis for sociocultural research. *Culture and Psychology*, 13(3), 307–32.

Morris, C. (2009) Developing pedagogy for doctors-as-teachers: the role of activity theory. In: H. Daniels, H. Lauder and J. Porter (eds) *Knowledge, Values and Educational Policy: a critical perspective*. London, Routledge, pp.273–81.

Norman, G. (2007) Editorial: how bad is medical education research anyway? *Advances in Health Science Education Theory and Practice*, 12(1), 1–5.

Postgraduate Medical Education and Training Board (PMETB) (2008) *Educating Tomorrow's Doctors: future models of medical training; medical workforce shape and trainee expectations*. Available from: www.gmc-uk.org/Educating_Tomorrows_Doctors_working_group_report_20080620_v1.pdf_30375087.pdf (accessed 2 January 2011).

Säljö, R. (2007) *Studying Learning and Knowing in Social Practices: units of analysis and tensions in theorising*. Lecture given on the occasion of the opening of The Oxford Centre for Socio-cultural Activity Theory Research, Oxford, UK. 14 March 2007.

Säljö, R. (2009) Learning, theories of learning, and units of analysis in research. *Educational Psychologist*, 44(3), 202–8.

Sfard, A. (1998) On two metaphors for learning and the dangers of choosing just one. *Educational Researcher*, 27(1), 4–13.

Swanwick, T. (2005) Informal learning in postgraduate medical education: from cognitivism to 'culturism'. *Medical Education*, 39(8), 859–65.

Teunissen, P. (2010) On the transfer of theory to the practice of research and education. *Medical Education*, 44(6), 534–5.

Tooke, J. (2007) *Aspiring to Excellence: findings and recommendations of the independent inquiry into modernising medical careers*, MMC Inquiry. Available at: www.mmcinquiry.org.uk/Final_8_Jan_08_MMC_all.pdf [last accessed 12 June 12].

Tooke, J. (2007) *Aspiring to Excellence: findings and recommendations of the independent inquiry into modernising medical careers*, MMC Inquiry.

Walton, J. and Steinert, Y. (2010) The anatomy of in-patient paediatric rounds: an observational study. *Medical Education*, 44(6), 550–8.

Wenger, E. (1998) *Communities of Practice: learning, meaning and identity*. Cambridge, Cambridge University Press.

2

Learning to teach on the job

Exploring the shape and significance of learning through work activity in medical settings

Viv Cook

> *The word 'doctor' means physician, and is derived from the Latin docere, to teach.*
>
> —Board of Medical Education

THE CONCEPT OF LEARNING THROUGH WORK ACTIVITY PROVIDES A critical lens with the potential to analyse and explore learning in clinical workplace settings. The study described in this chapter used theoretical and methodological tools that take account of and explore the influence of context on learning. It investigated how medical educators learn to teach in their place of work through their everyday practice, and thus the contexts included university lecture rooms, hospitals wards, theatres and general practice surgeries.

Doctors are required to teach other health professionals including junior members of their teams and students. The educational role of doctors has been given greater emphasis in recent years notably by the General Medical Council (2009, 1999) and the Board of Medical Education (2006). However, there is continuing debate about the most efficacious way in which doctors can be prepared to teach. Purcell and Lloyd-Jones (2003) point to the emergence of a 'plethora' (p.1) of short courses on teaching accompanied by longer programmes, observation of teaching and consultancy. While formal courses on how to teach play an important role, the focus of the research reported in this chapter was the informal learning to teach that takes place on the job.

This type of informal learning is sometimes also referred to as non-formal, work-based, workplace or experiential (I use these terms interchangeably except where otherwise stated); it is arguably crucial to professional development and yet lacks sufficient critical research attention. Researching this work-based 'on the job' evolution (McLeod *et al.*, 2006) can contribute to new models for faculty development beyond and in conjunction with formal provision. The study reported here aimed to make a contribution to understanding how doctors become med- ical educators. It was carried out as part of a doctorate completed by the author, delineating the work-based learning of novice teachers across hospital, general practice and university settings within one undergraduate London medical school – known for the purposes of the study as Central School (CS). The research asked: how and what do inexperienced medical educators learn about teaching on the job?

The research used theories and concepts that follow a socio-cultural perspect- ive on learning. Michael Eraut's (2004) theoretical understanding of learning through work activity and the concept of restrictive and expansive learning envi- ronments (Evans *et al.*, 2006) were used to explore the impact of contexts such as the realities and pressures of ward-based teaching experienced by junior doctors in their hospitals. Adopting a socio-cultural approach benefited the research by enabling an account of work-based learning to be told in which the challenges and complexities of teaching and learning in clinical working environments remained integral and also provided insights which were specific, relevant and finely tuned. It is argued that this allowed inferences to be drawn as to the relative opportun- ities for learning across university and clinical sites (to be referred to hereafter generically as 'medical settings').

Workplaces as sites for learning

The scale of work-based learning is aptly captured by Coffield's (2000) analogy of an 'iceberg', in which formal learning is just the tip, while informal learning, taking place in workplaces and communities, comprises the 'larger part hidden from view' (Cook, 2009, p.e608). This is not to suggest that there is a clear fixed distinction between 'informal' and 'formal' learning. Colley *et al.* (2002) pro- vide convincing argument that it is fruitless to base any analysis upon imagined boundaries between formal and informal (or non-formal), as learning takes place both in workplaces and educational institutions as an outcome of engagement and participation.

Theoretical approaches to investigating work-based learning have a long intellectual history. Hager (2010) charts the development from perspectives that focus largely upon psychological theories and the individual to those that emphasise a more socio-cultural view of learning. Socio-cultural approaches propose that learning takes place as a product of situated social activity (Lave and Wenger, 1991), an outcome of participation (Sfard, 1998) occurring within micro-social processes, shaped by cultural norms pertaining to and nuanced by individual workplaces mediated by a 'range of symbolic and conceptual tools' (Morris and Blaney, 2010, p.74). However, explanatory models of work-based learning still need to retain a balanced perspective that includes analysis at the level of the individual as well as context; one perspective should not divert attention from the other (Evans *et al.*, 2006). Eraut's work retains a strong commitment to the individual as a unit of analysis (Hager, 2010), but gives equal weight to the social context of learning, the social origins of knowledge and the cultural practices that realise knowledge in workplaces, stating that 'learning should be viewed through two lenses: the individual and the social' (Eraut, 2010, p.181). Eraut's theoretical approach was developed as a result of his research into early and mid-career learning in professional work, including healthcare (Eraut, 2010, 2004), and thus seemed particularly suitable for investigating and conceptualising the learning of medical educators.

How does work-based learning occur?

Eraut (2010) argues that work-based learning occurs as a 'by-product' of work activities, stemming naturally from the 'demands and challenges of work' (p.186), such as solving problems and 'trying things out'. Furthermore, he argues that learning is often achieved through the social activity of 'talking to other people' and is largely 'neither specific nor planned' (ibid.). Ellstrom (2010) makes a similar observation, that learning in the workplace is integral but subordinate to work practices and that it often occurs incidentally (also see Marsick and Watkins, 1990). Eraut (2010) also includes as work-based learning, short courses and mentoring (at or near the workplace) that have learning as a primary goal. However, I would argue that it is learning from key everyday work activity (bedside teaching, lectures, ward rounds, assessing students, attending meetings and so on) that should remain the key focus for research, if an innovative work-based learning agenda is to emerge for medical educators.

Eraut (2004) divides the activities of work-based learning into four categories: participation in group activities, working alongside others, tackling challenging tasks and working with clients. In all activities, the importance of context – social engagement with colleagues – is emphasised. This proposition finds resonance in other theoretical accounts – Lave and Wenger's (1991) seminal concept of legitimate peripheral participation foregrounds the centrality of 'working with others', while McNally *et al.* (2004), referring specifically to new teacher development, highlight the importance of workplace conversation.

Eraut (2004) also describes individual agency in learning through identifying actions such as observing, asking questions, listening, reflecting and learning from mistakes. Learning from work activities may occur with or without the intention to learn (Eraut, 2000; see also Ellstrom, 2010; Marsick and Watkins, 1990). It may occur implicitly, as a result of near spontaneous reaction or as a result of more planned deliberative reflection. Individual agency may account for variation in interest and commitment toward teaching within and between individual doctors. Additionally, whether a junior doctor or a lecturer on campus, the level of engagement that teachers have with their educational activities will be influenced by their job description, workload, routes for promotion and so on; 'the ways in which people learn in and through the workplace are rooted in educational trajectories and their complex intertwining with social institutions … at different stages in their life course' (Evans *et al.*, 2011a, p.356). Medical teachers bring their prior experiences of learning into their own beliefs about and practice of teaching as part of their internal frames of reference (Cairns and Malloch, 2010; Moon, 2004). As medical and educational professionals, they will be connected to a greater or lesser degree to wider continuing professional development networks in education – specialist subject centres, royal colleges, higher education academies, postgraduate centres – all of which colour and inform each individual's 'take' on professional life. Thus considerations of individual agency need to remain integral to any explanations of work-based learning.

What is being learnt in work-based learning?

The research undertaken at CS sought to understand not just *how* learning took place but also *what* was learnt. If Coffield's (2000) analogy is correct, then it

TABLE 2.1 A typology of 53 workplace learning trajectories

Task performance	**Role performance**
Speed and fluency	Prioritisation
Complexity of tasks and problems	Range of responsibility
Range of skills required	Supporting other people's learning
Communication with a range of people	Leadership
Collaborative work	Accountability
	Supervisory role
Awareness and understanding	Delegation
Other people: colleagues, customers, managers	Handling ethical issues
and so forth	Coping with unexpected problems
Contexts and situations	Crisis management
One's own organisation	Keeping up to date
Problems and risks	
Priorities and strategic issues	**Teamwork**
Value issues	Collaborative work
	Facilitating social relations
Personal development	Joint planning and problem-solving
Self-evaluation	Ability to engage in and promote mutual
Self-management	learning
Handling emotions	
Building and sustaining relationships	**Decision-making and problem-solving**
Disposition to attend to other perspectives	When to seek expert help
Disposition to consult and work with others	Dealing with complexity
Disposition to learn and improve one's practice	Group decision-making
Accessing relevant knowledge and expertise	Problem analysis
Ability to learn from experience	Formulating and evaluating options
	Managing the process within an appropriate
Academic knowledge and skills	timescale
Use of evidence and argument	Decision-making under pressure
Accessing formal knowledge	
Research-based practice	**Judgement**
Theoretical thinking	Quality of performance, output and outcome
Knowing what you might need to know	Priorities
Using knowledge resources (human, paper-	Value issues
based, electronic)	Levels of risk
Learning how to use relevant theory (in a range	
of practical situations)	

Source: Eraut *et al.* (2005:11)

seems reasonable to assume that the learning outcomes of work-based learning are considerable.

It has been argued that professional knowledge encompasses both public codified theory and knowledge about how to perform effectively – to get the job done. This distinction is also sometimes referred to as the difference between propositional or procedural knowledge – 'knowing that' and 'knowing how', or 'technical' and 'practical' knowledge (Beckett and Hager, 2002). More recently, these two dimensions have been supplemented by additional aspects of knowing, such as how to employ emotions within workplace relationships (Beatty, 2010). Professional knowledge is public and personal, codified and uncodified, practical and contextually related. To advance theory and practice, explanatory models of what is learnt must be employed that do not dichotomise but, rather, represent a blend, a 'variety of knowing' (Beckett and Hager, 2002) that reflects the complexity of performance. However, whichever model is adopted, it is important to avoid oversimplistic interpretations (Jenkins and Shipman, 1976) that do not do full justice to the complexity of work-based learning.

Eraut et al.'s (Eraut, 2004; Eraut et al., 2005; Eraut and Hirsch, 2007) typology of 'what' is being learnt in the workplace avoids oversimplification by identifying 53 workplace learning trajectories in eight categories (see Table 2.1). Eraut describes these trajectories as having authenticity in that they are 'readily recognisable' (2004, p.265) as products of work-based learning, based upon his previous research. The typology is offered as a research tool enabling investigators in the field to develop an understanding of learning trajectories in different professional contexts. The typology blends types of learning including skills, codified knowledge, dispositions and values. It encompasses a sense of the dynamic of work-based learning through the expectation that individuals will travel at different rates along these trajectories during their lives. In summary, the typology offers an open-ended exploratory tool originating from research on work-based learning that can be used to generate the form, colour and shape of the learning that may occur in different professional contexts.

Medical settings as sites for learning: degrees of expansiveness

Eraut (2004) proposes that collaborative work activity is a basis for learning. It follows naturally from this to question the degree to which workplaces afford opportunities for participation in activities that lead to learning – to 'acquire expertise' (Evans et al., 2006, p.43). The degree to which individuals are able or allowed to learn in their places of work is given greater prominence in some accounts of work-based learning than others; notably, for example, foregrounded in the work of Stephen Billett (2010, 2004) in his exposition of workplace 'affordances' and in the use by Evans *et al.* (2006) of the concept of workplace 'expansiveness'.

From their empirical data on work-based learning in a range of different contexts, Evans *et al.* (2006) constructed a framework for analysing the expansiveness of learning environments. This extended Lave and Wenger's (1991) concept of community of practice to give a greater focus upon 'access to forms of participation and work organisation' (p.36). They demonstrated application of the framework by presenting nine key *features* of expansive and restrictive learning environments for secondary school teachers (see figure 3.1 in Evans *et al.*, 2006, p.53) identified in research conducted by Hodkinson and Hodkinson (2003). These features are highly congruent with the view that learning in the workplace, in this instance teaching, takes place largely as by-product of work activity in ways that are largely social and interactive (as in Eraut's analysis). For the purposes of my research, the specific features of expansive learning environments for teachers were adapted to apply to on-campus (university), hospital and general practice settings. This meant excluding features that implied the status of teaching as the primary activity within the workplace environment, for example, an excluded item was 'an explicit focus on teacher learning as a dimension of normal working practices' (Evans, 2006, p.53). Put simply, clinical work (and not teaching) is the main activity in hospitals and general practices. This process of exclusion resulted in five relevant remaining features, which were synthesised and adapted to medical settings (*see* Box 2.1). These features were used to review collections of individual accounts of work-based learning so that inferences could be drawn about the relative expansiveness of settings across CS.

Box 2.1 Features of expansive learning environments used in the research

- Close collaborative working (co-tutor; opportunities to observe, to be observed and to receive feedback)
- Exposure to a wide range of educational activities
- Opportunities to teach in a wide range of environments
- Opportunities for networking outside the immediate environment
- Personal needs in teaching identified and development supported

---

Work-based learning of novice teachers: the study in further detail

The research study set out to map the contours of the work-based learning of novice medical educators across medical settings, including on-campus and clinical sites, which collectively comprise CS medical school. The aim was to delineate both *what* and *how* work-based learning took place and to make comparisons across medical settings in terms of the opportunities they afforded for learning – their expansiveness. Full details of the study are published elsewhere (see Cook, 2009) – for the purposes of this chapter, what follows is a summary of the method and outcomes to enable evaluation of the adoption of a socio-cultural approach to exploring the work-based learning of clinical teachers.

Twelve novice teachers (with fewer than 3 years' teaching experience or with teaching as a minor role) were recruited for interview. The focus was on inexperienced faculty since the early years of teaching are a key developmental period (Knight, 2002; Eraut, 1994) and thus likely to be particularly illuminative of workplace learning. The participants were drawn from the three teaching sites at CS – on campus, in general practice and/or in hospital settings. By means of open-ended and exploratory questions, they were invited to narrate their own workplace learning, describing the colleagues and events that were pivotal to their progress as educators. They were encouraged to think across all their main work activities and to try also to capture and relate smaller, more incidental, more surprising and 'out of the ordinary' events that gave rise to learning. The typology of Eraut (2004) (*see* Table 2.1 for Eraut *et al.* 2005 version) of what is being learnt was used as the primary analytical tool together with a model denoting features of expansive learning environments (*see* Box 2.1). To support verification of their accounts (Miles and Huberman, 1994), the participants were invited to comment on the outcomes of the analysis through the use of a written summary of the main themes presented back to them in story form.

A key consideration in conducting the interviews was that work-based learning is often tacit in nature (Nonaka and Takeuchi, 1995; Molander, 1992). Knowledge gained is often an integral part of routine professional skills and expertise, aptly captured in Polanyi's famous description, 'that which we know but cannot tell' (1967). It is questionable whether individuals can identify and characterise their own learning in ways that can be articulated (*see* Chapter 6 by Mary Gobbi for further discussion on conceptualising 'the tacit'). To aid elicitation of the tacit dimension of learning, two strategies were adopted. First, in line with previous research (Eraut *et al.*, 1998), all participants were interviewed twice, thus allowing them an intervening period of 3–4 months to reflect on the nature of their workplace learning. The second strategy was to use a concept map to help participants visualise and project their learning through work activity. Hakim (1987) posits that specialised techniques are often needed to elicit 'aspects of respondent's views that are not directly articulated' (p.27). Such techniques may include repertory grids (based upon personal constructs) (Kelly, 1955) or techniques to facilitate the projection of ideas, including picture or sentence completion. In this instance, a concept 'map' was used as the primary technique. This method of data collection has been previously employed to elicit teachers' conceptual understanding of organisational changes in their workplaces (Khattri and Miles, 1993). Novak and Cañas (2006) describe concept maps in the following way:

> [U]sually enclosed in circles or boxes of some type and relationships between concepts indicated by a connecting line linking two concepts. Words on the line, referred to as linking words or linking phrases, specify the relationship between the two concepts. (p.1)

A simple outline of a concept map was constructed (*see* Figure 2.1), which participants were invited to complete during the course of the interview. Its design conformed to Novak and Cañas's (2006) description in that it allowed participants to signify the relationship between aspects of their concepts about the subject to be explored: in this instance, learning. Two items represented Eraut's (2004) fourfold classification of how people learn at work: people and tasks. The concept map was used to help participants reconstruct their learning experiences in the space of a short interview. The consistent use of people and tasks as organising categories with participants from different medical settings in CS also facilitated comparisons across these settings.

Participants were encouraged to view themselves on a journey of development in their places of work. To aid them, an upward arrow was placed in the centre of the map utilising Dreyfus and Dreyfus's (1986) concepts of novice and expert, which were placed at either end. They were asked to write the names of people and tasks that were most influential in their learning and development in the circles on the map. They were asked to put those most important to them closest to the arrow. They were required to identify learning from work activities, but, unsurprisingly, some drew in more planned learning events such as formal courses.

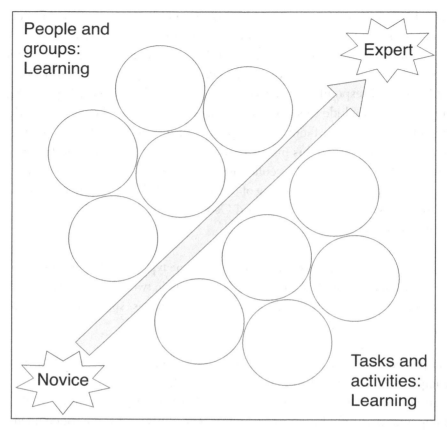

People and groups: Learning

Expert

Novice

Tasks and activities: Learning

FIGURE 2.1 Interview concept map (from Cook (2009) © 2009 Informa Healthcare; reproduced with permission of Informa Healthcare)

Some findings: the how, what and where of work-based learning

The results reported in this chapter focus on the analysis of *what* was being learnt, as an exemplar of one type of socio-cultural approach to research. However, it is worth noting that informal collaborative work-based learning was the main feature of participants' accounts of *how* learning took place in the form of observing colleagues' practice, co-tutoring and networking at internal and external events.

In terms of *what* was being learnt, four headings from the typology of learning trajectories by Eraut (2004) were most commonly used to code data from the interviews and maps. These four headings, together with examples of emergent descriptors, are set out in Figure 2.2.

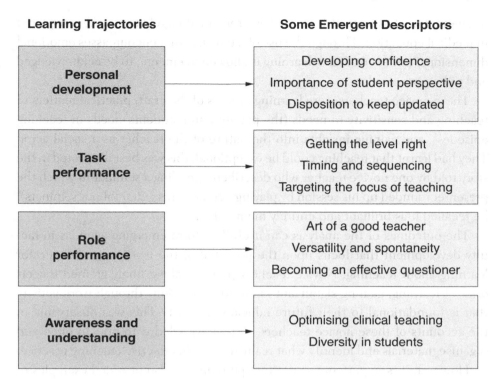

Learning Trajectories   **Some Emergent Descriptors**

Personal development	Developing confidence Importance of student perspective Disposition to keep updated
Task performance	Getting the level right Timing and sequencing Targeting the focus of teaching
Role performance	Art of a good teacher Versatility and spontaneity Becoming an effective questioner
Awareness and understanding	Optimising clinical teaching Diversity in students

FIGURE 2.2 What is being learnt by novice teachers? (from Cook (2009) © 2009 Informa Healthcare; adapted with permission of Informa Healthcare)

Novice teachers were learning about role and task performance, personal development, and awareness and understanding. Unsurprisingly, they were learning the nuts and bolts of planning and delivering teaching, but also about themselves and others as teachers. There were some rather more unexpected findings – namely, the importance of learning confidence. Although gaining confidence might be expected to be a key aspect of work-based learning, what was surprising was the level of emotional challenge in teaching for some of these novice teachers. For example, they were learning to handle fears about being centre stage in a lecture theatre presenting to a large audience of medical students. In a similar way, junior doctors were learning to deal with their fears regarding the limits of their clinical knowledge when teaching on the wards:

> I'm still a bit insecure about my own knowledge … 'cause I'm still learning myself, so you know, I don't want to say the wrong things. Some students can be really knowledgeable and … sometimes you feel like they know everything already. (Case 8: junior doctor, hospital)

Such emotional aspects of learning have remained largely tacit and unexplored in medical education. Through the use of a typology that encompasses emotional dimensions, evidence of such learning is allowed to emerge, to be acknowledged and to be given credence.

These novice teachers were learning aspects of the craft, practical matters of teaching and sensitivity to needs (the patients' and students' needs in teaching episodes), and gaining insights into the nature of the teacher as a social actor. They had learnt that teaching could be exceptional; this was best illustrated in the story told by one novice teacher who described attending a seminar in which the presenter rounded up his session by playing a song on his guitar (about seminars); he recalled it as brilliant and entirely memorable.

The outcomes of the analysis can usefully inform emerging agendas in faculty development that focus upon the potential of the workplace as a site for learning about teaching. Novice teachers progress along finely grained trajectories of learning, gaining significant knowledge and skills through work activity that is foundational to their future educational work. This was observable in the accounts of these novice teachers, as they wrestled with how to pitch and organise materials and identify what really matters in effective teaching practice.

However, it is important to note that participants also provided examples of observing work-based teaching behaviour that was suboptimal:

> [T]hey [senior doctors] feel they have to do it because they need to tick a box, essentially it's negligible what the benefit is to both sides, because they're not really getting anything out of it and the student's kind of just sitting there, hearing about it. (Case 8: junior doctor, hospital)

In this case, the junior doctor learnt something positive: that it is important to be motivated and that 'tick-boxing' is evident to the learner. Nevertheless, there is a message here of professional importance, that the approaches taken and outcomes of work-based learning can be undesirable.

Results suggested that opportunities for work-based learning varied between the medical settings in CS. This is illustrated by one general practitioner who said she felt she was somewhat restricted in her learning because of the small amount of teaching that she did and repeated each year: 'Most of the time I would like to do more teaching but it is difficult – you need to put yourself forward much more to get teaching' (Case 11). However, this should not necessarily be interpreted as meaning that some medical settings provided more expansive learning environments than others. The pervading influence of individual agency in the form of competing priorities (research and clinical) often emerged in the interviews as important overriding factors influencing the different levels of engagement and learning in the medical educator role.

Some methodological insights: typologies, maps and features

This was a complex study that explored the very broad and interwoven fabric of the work-based learning of novice teachers in different medical settings. The conceptual approach used recognised learning as something arising from work activity: a result of individual and collaborative activity shaped by the workplace environment. The design and conduct of the study yielded some interesting methodological insights on using a preset typology of *what* is being learnt, using concept 'maps' to elicit telling, and using the concept of features of expansiveness to review and compare learning, each of which are considered in more detail later in this chapter.

The typology of Eraut and his colleagues (Eraut, 2004; Eraut *et al.*, 2005; Eraut & Hirsch 2007) concerning what is being learnt was developed as a research tool for capturing the broad essence and nature of workplace learning. In practice, the learning trajectories did provide an effective starting point for coding data. Evidence of learning as a result of work-based activities was observable in participants' accounts across headings such as role and task performance. The typology's usefulness as a tool is borne out by the similarities in the outcomes from coding in terms of 'what' was being learnt with other studies of medical educators (MacDougall and Drummond, 2005; Mann *et al.*, 2001). Using the typology requires interpretation and translation into contextually appropriate descriptors for coding. In this study, this meant generating descriptors that reflected teaching activity in medical settings. For example, 'contexts and situations' became about 'optimising clinical teaching', with coded data relating to 'working with patients'.

In this study, the typology was used to interpret accounts of learning collected through individual narratives. It might be argued that using the typology in this way, i.e. categorising the self-reported learning of participants, risks the creation of an idealistic non-contextual account of learning achieved. Research in the field needs to enable learning to be framed and assessed within the context in which it takes place. More recently, Eraut (2010) describes using points on the learning trajectories as 'windows on episodes of practice', in which features of whole performance and its antecedents need to be taken into account in determining whether learning has been sustained or enhanced. This will require the researcher to employ methods that enable the capture of individual performance and its context in fine detail – for example, through observation of work activity and learning.

On a further note, it has been argued that there is a need to use approaches that move beyond understanding what is learnt through categorising learning claims, to a concern with how knowledge is put to work and how its features are played out and recontextualised in different settings (Evans *et al.*, 2011b). A focus upon the process of 'pedagogic recontextualisation' (p.156), how disciplinary knowledge and practice-based knowledge are combined by educators as they organise learning activities, offers further possibilities for researching the practice of clinical teaching.

The completion of the concept maps provided a rich source of data. They triggered participants' understanding of the nature of the research and provided a focused moment in the first interview to think about their own places of work. Meaningful insights were generated as participants identified exactly which people and tasks were most significant to their learning. The arrow placed in the centre of the map provided an opportunity for them to assess their progress as an educator to date, and this led them to recognise that some areas of their skills were more advanced than others. This latter point is significant, since one potential limitation of using an upward arrow to represent the stage of learning is that it suggests that development is linear and 'across the board'; in the event, such one-dimensional thinking was not evident in participants' accounts. For example, they would claim that they were a better clinical skills teacher than a classroom lecturer. Participants recognised that they were progressing along some learning trajectories while stalling in others. Completing the map helped them to round out and elaborate their accounts. It was in the course of completing the maps that the multidimensional influences on work-based learning really came into view. Within the space of a few moments, they would refer to their experiences of working with colleagues, everyday tasks, observations and personal histories. The maps also revealed a good deal about the intricacies of different clinical settings – the working arrangements, spheres of activity and contact with others outside their immediate environment. For this reason, the maps, which were used to elicit the tacit and the hidden within an interview process, might be given further prominence as a research tool in exploring learning through narrative accounts. This could be achieved by spending further time focusing upon the contours of the maps, the nature of their completion and their symbolic importance to the participant.

Finally, the concept of expansiveness was utilised to explore the realities and differences of working and learning in different medical settings by means of a five-feature model (*see* Box 2.1). The five features did facilitate distinction, with commonalities and differences emerging across sites that may be of some professional significance. However, a cautionary note is needed before drawing any conclusions with respect to settings. Specifically, while it might have been possible to indicate that some workplaces seemed to offer fewer opportunities for work-based learning, this should be measured against the needs, roles and current trajectories of individuals. Having greater opportunities to expand their teaching load or take part in further networking may not have fitted the needs of some medical educators who had other professional roles, such as junior doctors fully engaged with clinical tasks. If meaningful assessments are to be made about work-based learning and the relative expansiveness of different clinical environments, then individual agency and the social context of the workplace need to be considered in tandem in the process of analysis.

In conclusion, the study findings suggested that work-based learning plays a considerable role in the professional development of novice medical educators. The study demonstrated that such learning can be effectively explored though a conceptual lens that characterises work-based learning as integral to individual and collaborative action shaped by professional context. The study also illustrated how the use of a generic typology of learning trajectories can be used to inform analysis of potential learning and may have additional value in highlighting aspects of learning that have hitherto received minimal attention, such as handling emotions. Research that fosters articulation of the tacit, the informal and the unrecognised aspects of learning has the potential to validate learning experiences and facilitate development for those who engage as research participants, as well as to inform faculty development. However, such learning should be viewed critically. If work-based learning is to be part of the spectrum of faculty development, then it should be acknowledged that it can be undesirable as well as desirable, and self-affirming as well as born from the insights gained from reflection. By its nature, such learning will be variable and inconsistent. Most importantly, if the potential of learning through work activity is to be enhanced, then its relationship with other types of learning along the continuum of formality, including planned programmes of learning, needs to be understood in much greater detail.

Acknowledgements

This chapter is based on work carried out by the author and was previously reported in 2009 (see Cook, 2009). Thanks to the Centre for Excellence in Work-based Learning, based at the Institute of Education, University of London who funded the research and Professor Michael Eraut who gave permission to reproduce the typology (2005).

References

Beatty, B. (2010) Seeing workplace learning through an emotional lens. In: M. Malloch, L. Cairns, K. Evans, *et al.* (eds) *The Sage Handbook of Workplace Learning*. London, Sage, pp.341–55.

Beckett, D. and Hager, P. (2002) *Life, Work and Learning: practice in postmodernity*. New York, NY, Routledge.

Billett, S. (2004) Learning through work: workplace participatory practices. In: H. Rainbird, A. Fuller and A. Munro (eds) *Workplace Learning in Context*. London, Routledge, pp.109–25.

Billett, S. (2010) Subjectivity, self and personal agency in learning though and for work. In: M. Malloch, L. Cairns, K. Evans, *et al.* (eds) *The Sage Handbook of Workplace Learning*. London, Sage, pp.60–72.

Board of Medical Education (2006) *Doctors as Teachers*. London, British Medical Association.

Cairns, L. and Malloch, M. (2010) Theories of work, place and learning: new directions. In: M. Malloch, L. Cairns, K. Evans, *et al.* (eds) *The Sage Handbook of Workplace Learning*. London, Sage, pp.3–16.

Coffield, F. (ed.) (2000) *The Necessity of Informal Learning*. Bristol, Policy Press in association with the ESRC Learning Society Programme.

Colley, H., Hodkinson P. and Malcolm J. (2002) *Non-formal Learning: mapping the conceptual terrain*. Available from: www.infed.org/archives/e-texts/colley_informal_learning.htm (accessed 26 October 2010).

Cook, V. (2009) Mapping the work-based learning of novice teachers: charting some rich terrain. *Medical Teacher*, 31(12), e608–14.

Dreyfus, H. L. and Dreyfus, S. E. (1986) *Mind Over Machine: the power of human intuition and expertise in the era of the computer*. Oxford, Basil Blackwell.

Ellstrom, P. (2010) Informal learning at work: conditions, processes and logics. In: M. Malloch, L. Cairns, K. Evans, *et al.* (eds) *The Sage Handbook of Workplace Learning*. London, Sage, pp.105–19.

Eraut, M. (1994) *Developing Professional Knowledge and Competence*. London, Falmer Press.

Eraut, M. (2004) Informal learning in the workplace. *Studies in Continuing Education*, 26(2), 247–73.

Eraut, M. (2010) How researching learning at work can lead to tools for enhancing learning. In: M. Malloch, L. Cairns, K. Evans, *et al.* (eds) *The Sage Handbook of Workplace Learning*. London, Sage, pp.181–97.

Eraut, M., Alderton J., Cole G., *et al.* (1998) Learning from other people at work. In: F. Coffield (ed.) *Learning at Work: the learning society*. Bristol, Policy Press, pp.37–48.

Eraut M. and Hirsch W. (2007) The significance of workplace learning for individuals, groups and organisation. SKOPE monograph. University of Oxford, Department of Economics.

Eraut, M., Maillardet, F., and Miller, C., *et al.* (2005) What is learned in the workplace and how? Typologies and results from a cross-professional longitudinal study. Presented at the EARLI Biannual Conference, Nicosia, 23–27 August.

Evans, K., Hodkinson, P., Rainbird, H., *et al.* (2006) *Improving Workplace Learning*. London, Routledge.

Evans, K., Waite E. and Kersh N. (2011a) Towards a social ecology of adult learning in and through the workplace. In: M. Malloch, L. Cairns, K. Evans, *et al.* (eds) *The Sage Handbook of Workplace Learning*. London, Sage, pp.356–72.

Evans, K., Guile D. and Harris J. (2011b) Rethinking work-based learning: for education professionals and professionals who educate. In: M. Malloch, L. Cairns, K. Evans, *et al.* (eds) *The Sage Handbook of Workplace Learning*. London, Sage, pp.149–61.

General Medical Council (GMC) (1999) *The Doctor as Teacher*. London, GMC.

General Medical Council (GMC) (2009) *Tomorrow's Doctors*. London, GMC.

Hager, P. (2010) Theories of workplace learning. In: M. Malloch, L. Cairns, K. Evans, *et al.* (eds) *The Sage Handbook of Workplace Learning*. London, Sage, pp.17–31.

Hakim, C. (1987) *Research Design: strategies and choices in the design of social research*. London, Allen & Unwin.

Hodkinson, P. and Hodkinson, H. (2003) Individuals, communities of practice and the policy context: school-teachers learning in their workplace. *Studies in Continuing Learning*, 25(1), 3–21.

Jenkins, D. and Shipman, M. D. (1976) *Curriculum: an introduction*. London, Open Books Publishing.

Kelly, G. A. (1955) *The Psychology of Personal Constructs*. New York, NY, Norton.

Khattri, N. and Miles, M. B. (1993) *Mapping Restructuring*. Final technical report. New York, NY, Centre for Policy Research.

Knight, P. (2002) *Being a Teacher in Higher Education*. Buckingham, Society for Research into Higher Education and Open University Press.

Lave, J. and Wenger, E. (1991) *Situated Learning: legitimate peripheral participation*. Cambridge, Cambridge University Press.

MacDougall, J. and Drummond, M. J. (2005) The development of medical teachers: an enquiry into the learning histories of 10 experienced medical teachers. *Medical Education*, 39(12), 1213–20.

Mann, K. V., Holmes, D. B., Hayes, V. M., *et al.* (2001) Community family medicine teachers' perceptions of their teaching role. *Medical Education*, 35(3), 278–85.

Marsick, V. J. and Watkins, K. (1990) *Informal and Incidental Learning in the Workplace*. New York, NY, Routledge.

McLeod, P. J., Steinert, Y., Meagher, T., *et al.* (2006) The acquisition of tacit knowledge in medical education: learning by doing. *Medical Education*, 40(2), 146–9.

McNally, J., Boreham, N., Cope, P., *et al.* (2004) Informal learning in early teacher development. Draft of paper presented at the BERA Conference, Manchester, 14–18 September. Available from: www.leeds.ac.uk/educol/documents/00003933.pdf (accessed 12 July 2010).

Miles, M. B. and Huberman, M. A. (1994) *Qualitative Data Analysis.* 2nd edn. London, Sage.

Molander, B. (1992) Tacit knowledge and silenced knowledge: fundamental problems and controversies. In: B. Goranzon and M. Florin (eds) *Skill and Education: reflection and experience.* London, Springer-Verlag, pp.9–31.

Moon, J. A. (2004) *A Handbook of Reflective and Experiential Learning: theory and practice.* London, RoutledgeFalmer.

Morris, C. and Blaney, D. (2010) Work-based learning. In: T. Swanwick (ed.) *Understanding Medical Education.* Edinburgh and Chichester, ASME and Wiley-Blackwell, pp.69–82.

Nonaka, I. and Takeuchi, A. (1995) *The Knowledge Creating Company: how Japanese companies create the dynamics of innovation.* New York, NY, Oxford University Press.

Novak, J. D. and Cañas, J. (2006) *The Theory Underlying Concept Maps and How to Construct Them.* Florida Institute for Human and Machine Cognition (IHMC). Available from: http://cmap.ihmc.us/Publications/ResearchPapers/TheoryCmaps/TheoryUnderlyingConceptMaps.htm (accessed 18 January 2007).

Polanyi, M. (1967) *The Tacit Dimension.* Garden City, NY, Doubleday.

Purcell, N. and Lloyd-Jones, G. (2003) Standards for medical educators. *Medical Education*, 37(2), 149–54.

Sfard, A. (1998) On two metaphors of learning for learning and the dangers of choosing just one. *Educational Researcher*, 27(1), 4–13.

3

Assessment in natural settings in obstetrics and gynaecology

Insights from a guided learning perspective

Vikram Jha, Zeryab Setna and Trudie Roberts

Introduction

The association between learning and assessment in the workplace is an important one (Billett, 2000). The development of professional expertise and competence in professions occurs primarily in the workplace. Novice trainees acquire the knowledge and skills required to become independent practitioners by working alongside and learning from their peers and seniors. As training progresses, supervisors are able to informally observe trainees performing the required tasks and demonstrating their experiential learning. Based on several such observations, over time, supervisors are able to make an overall judgement on competence. These assessment processes occurring alongside routine work are not necessarily unstructured; however, they are implicit and often left unrecorded (van der Vleuten, 1996). Over the last decade, however, assessment has become more formalised and structured in a number of specialisms, including medicine, through the introduction of a wide range of workplace assessment methods.

This chapter explores how learning can take place alongside and as a result of assessment in the workplace. Underpinning this exploration is a theoretical framework suggested for effective learning in the workplace: the development of expertise through learning at work (Billett, 2001, 1999, 1996). This framework allows exploration of how people develop professional competence through performance of routine and non-routine tasks in the workplace, guided by their supervisors, and through transitions from less accountable to more accountable tasks. Implicitly linked with Billett's framework is Piaget's (1996) theory of cognitive development, particularly with regard to the way cognitive functioning processes are adapted during transition from novice to expert. In addition, with the focus of this chapter being on assessment, van der Vleuten's (1996) conceptualisation of professional competence and its assessment also provides a crucial conceptual link with Billett's framework. This chapter is divided into four sections. In the first section, the strategies suggested by Billett are discussed, along with their implicit links with Piaget's theory of cognitive development and van der Vleuten's conceptualisation of professional competence. The second section provides an overview of a research programme on learning in the context of workplace assessment. Relevant results from this research are discussed in the third section in the light of Billett's framework. The chapter concludes with a summary of the advantages of using such a framework, the challenges of research in this area and suggestions for future research.

The development of expertise through learning at work: cognitive structures, context specificity and guided learning

Billett (2000) posits a model of workplace learning in which learning is conceptualised as a 'product of everyday thinking and acting' and includes learning that occurs during the course of routine daily work. In most professions, he argues, people try to make sense of situations that they encounter during their day-to-day work (Billett, 2000), often learning to perform tasks by problem-solving and making adaptations to their cognitive structures (Piaget, 1966). The problems encountered may be related to routine tasks, i.e. something that we do at work several times a day, or more non-routine tasks, i.e. something that we do only occasionally, when a new responsibility or situation presents itself. However, according to Billett, the development of cognitive structures and skills acquisition through carrying out routine work activities alone has some limitations. First, each workplace has its own norms regarding the type of work performed and how it is performed. Second, there are issues with hierarchical structures within organisations, including division of tasks and accountability to different people.

This 'hidden curriculum' has the potential to exert considerable influence on what is learnt and how it is learnt. Some of the outcomes from this hidden curriculum may be undesirable, for example taking shortcuts, or replicating unprofessional behaviour observed from role models (Billett, 1996).

In Billett's scheme, learning at work occurs not through conducting the usual work tasks alone, but in combination with close supervision and guidance from colleagues and experts (Billett, 1996). He furthers this notion of learning at work by suggesting that by performing routine work and through guidance from colleagues, the novice learners gradually begin to develop their expertise and start to move from simple tasks with low accountability to more complex tasks with higher accountability. Simultaneously, there is a tendency for learners to move from peripheral to full participation in non-routine and difficult tasks as they evolve as experts in the workplace, as first suggested by Lave and Wenger (1991). This participation is not always a stepwise sequence, but rather involves groups of activities that are observed and then performed, depending on when they arise at the workplace.

In medicine, learners at the start of their training often have to perform basic and less accountable tasks, such as clerking-in patients, taking blood samples, following up results and observing and assisting at procedures. As they gain experience, these tasks change to more accountable ones such as performing procedures under guidance and becoming more responsible for the delivery of patient management. As senior trainees, on the threshold of becoming experts, they begin to take responsibility for tasks such as performing procedures independently, making diagnostic decisions and organising and implementing management plans. This development of expertise and transition from novice to expert is in keeping with Lave and Wenger's (1991) concept of professional expertise development and overlaps with Piaget's (1966) theory in ways later described. Gaining confidence and becoming more competent depends on the exposure to clinical complexity that the workplace offers to the individual trainee.

Billett's proposition that learning goes hand-in-hand with work activity is similar in some respects to aspects of Piaget's (1966) theory of cognitive development, particularly with regard to the way cognitive functioning processes are adapted during transition from novice to expert. Although originally developed to study cognitive development in children, Piaget's theory finds application in adult education and workplace learning equally well (Billett, 1999). Cognitive functioning, according to Piaget (1966), refers to the processes that account for changes in the cognitive structure according to different situations or conditions.

He uses the terms 'organisation' and 'adaptation' to explain how the cognitive structure may be changed by an individual while maintaining its integrity. Organisation, used to explain increasing complexity of actions and thought processes as an individual develops, is the ability to integrate actions into coherent structures to result in higher order activity. This allows for a 'continuity of cognitive structure across time and development' (Bybee and Sund, 1982). Adaptation refers to the tendency of people to adjust to their environment, for example when faced with an unfamiliar situation or task. This implies that their cognitive structure may change, depending on adaptations that the individual makes according to the environment. Adaptation has two main components: assimilation and accommodation. During assimilation, the individual makes sense of a situation by modifying it to fit their existing cognitive structure. Accommodation, on the other hand, requires a change in existing cognitive structure or explanation to make sense of a situation, i.e. structures are broadened or expanded to make sense of increasing numbers and complexities of situations in the environment.

Billett's model of how learners achieve expertise at work is congruent with another widely used model of professional competence described by van der Vleuten (1996). The traditional trait model of competence was based on an individual's personal component attributes that developed over time until competence was achieved. These component attributes were also considered to be relatively stable across work situations and time frames and it was assumed that gaining expertise in one work area or skill allowed individuals to perform professionally across all situations. Van der Vleuten (1996) offers a revised perspective of competence. He suggests that different components of competence tend to vary depending upon the nature of the task performed, and expertise in one type of skill does not necessarily translate to expertise in another. This view resonates with Billett's explanation that the performance of even routine tasks is often contextual and may vary depending upon the structure and culture of individual workplaces. It also links in with the concept of 'content specificity' first suggested by Elstein *et al.* (1978) and used to explain why performances vary from one problem to another (Eva *et al.*, 1998). Generally speaking, correlation between individual performances is low because the content of different tasks varies and performance depends on how familiar individual performers are with this content. In addition, the development of competence depends initially on the acquisition of relevant knowledge, with experts being more capable of accessing and applying knowledge to challenging situations than novice learners, an idea similar to Piaget's (1966) accommodation. This knowledge is best used when it is acquired and stored in an appropriate context in relation to the nature of the task and circumstances under which it was performed. With increasing expertise, however, clinical reasoning no longer depends entirely on cognitive processes, but also uses intuitive and automated processes developed as a result of experience in the workplace.

In Billett's framework, guidance by experts is a major factor that determines learners' ability to acquire adequate knowledge and expertise to perform tasks in the workplace. Although guidance at work may adopt various forms including mentoring individuals over periods of time, assisting new learners to perform unfamiliar tasks or acting as role models of acceptable professional behaviour (Garvey, 1994; Gay, 1994), the type of guidance Billett focuses on in his framework 'involves more experienced or expert workers assisting in the development of the vocational practice of less experienced workers' (Billett, 2001, p.141). According to Billett, three levels of guidance may occur. We discuss these levels here using Billett's perspectives, but in the context of medicine.

Level 1: organising and managing learners' experiences in the workplace

This first level, according to Billett, involves creating a curriculum and opportunities at the workplace for learners to perform the tasks required for them to progress within the profession. In our experience in medicine, this involves the identification of core competencies that should be acquired at progressive stages of training. This notion of a curriculum for trainee doctors is a relatively new concept; prior to this, the unstructured training did not necessarily provide guidance on the competencies to be attained by the end of training. During routine work, clinical encounters that allow display of these competencies are identified by learners or supervisors and form the basis of assessment. Supervisors can monitor the initiative and drive demonstrated by learners in wanting to move from the previously described peripheral to full participation in both routine and non-routine tasks. The onus for learning and assessment is therefore a shared one, with both learners and supervisors adopting responsibility for this.

Level 2: guidance in the development of procedures and understanding associated with work practice

The second level of guidance in Billett's framework requires trainers to model key tasks and demonstrate procedures for the benefit of learners. This also involves coaching trainees in these tasks and sharing knowledge and skills that could not be accessed without the input from experts. This is particularly applicable to relatively novice learners. At this level of guidance, trainees may need to be regularly assessed formatively, performing procedures and managing cases under direct and (later) indirect supervision by experts.

Level 3: development of self-regulated learning and ability to transfer knowledge and skills to other workplaces

This final level involves engaging trainees in reflecting on what they have learnt, providing them with feedback on their performance compared with both their peers and the standards expected at their level of training. It also allows for discussion regarding transferability of skills and knowledge acquired to different work settings. It is the responsibility of the expert trainers to ensure that the learner acquires knowledge that is not only sufficient to perform that particular task but also, and more important, transferable to other tasks and settings relevant to the profession. This is not always the case in practice, as some trainers may be reluctant teachers, or they may feel concerned about being displaced or outshone by their juniors (Lave and Wenger, 1991).

Billett's analysis and perspective on workplace learning in respect to the centrality of guided supervision holds value for evaluating the learning arising from assessment regimes within specialty training in medicine across the world. Their potential effectiveness is impacted upon by the realities of the clinical context. Despite a drive toward senior-led service in a number of specialties, the majority of out-of-hours service is still provided by doctors in training (Temple, 2010). A significant proportion of learning opportunities are encountered during routine service provision, i.e. when carrying out routine clinical tasks, but often without the guidance of senior staff. The delivery of clinical services has also changed in the last decade, with greater emphasis on achieving targets such as waiting times and increasing turnover of clinical activity. This has made direct supervision of trainees in high-pressure clinical areas such as outpatient clinics and operating theatres challenging. Consequently, one concern is that the potential for learning may not be realised since there is insufficient guidance and assisted reflection to enable development though assessment.

Research evaluating learning in the context of workplace assessment

More formalised workplace assessment processes have developed in professional education to allow trainees to be observed and assessed in naturalistic settings. These processes are meant to lay emphasis on the formative assessment of trainees with feedback on performance and formulation of action plans for future learning. A major focus of workplace assessment should, therefore, be on facilitation of learning rather than only being a test of competence. However, in some professions, including medicine, there is a culture of adopting assessment methods with a focus on assessment alone, with less regard to ascertaining the learning that is taking place alongside assessment (Setna *et al.*, 2010).

We were commissioned by the Royal College of Obstetricians and Gynaecologists to evaluate the implementation of workplace-based assessment as part of training within the specialty. Three types of assessment methods allow direct observation of specific individual clinical encounters: (1) objective structured assessment of technical skills (OSATS), (2) mini-clinical evaluation exercise (mini-CEX) and (3) case-based discussion (CbD). A summary of these methods and the competency domains they assess is provided in Table 3.1.

TABLE 3.1 Types of assessment and their competency domains

Type of form	Domains assessed
Mini-clinical evaluation exercise	Six clinical domains: (1) history taking, (2) physical examination skills, (3) communication skills, (4) clinical judgement, (5) professionalism and (6) organisation and efficiency Also marks for overall clinical competence
Objective structured assessment of technical skills	Two components: (1) a checklist of specific competencies required to perform a particular procedure and (2) a generic skills form that measures more generic competencies such as tissue or instrument handling and communication with the team
Case-based discussion	Four domains: (1) medical record keeping, (2) clinical assessment, (3) decision-making and (4) professionalism

It is our experience that trainees learning to become independent practitioners within the specialty perform numerous routine and non-routine tasks in diverse clinical settings. Novice learners would initially mostly observe senior colleagues performing these tasks, and would then start carrying out some of them under direct supervision. As learners move from peripheral to more central participation, they will begin to perform a number of these procedures or tasks under indirect supervision or finally independently. This gradual development of competence through learning while working is similar to other professions such as coal mining (Billett, 1993) or tailoring (Lave, 1990).

The assessment methods described earlier have been designed to allow these performances to be observed and formally evaluated by senior colleagues.

A clinical task is carried out either under direct supervision of the senior colleague or independently under direct observation. This depends on the expectations of the level of competence of the trainee and the complexity of the task. In practice, supervisors or learners select specific clinical encounters that they feel should be formally assessed. This depends largely on the availability of senior colleagues to observe and assess these performances. As mentioned earlier, a good deal of routine service provision, particularly outside regular working hours, occurs in the absence of senior consultant supervision. This places limits on assessment, since it can only take place when both trainees and seniors are available together. Assessment could be in any of the domains described in Table 3.1, with the performance assessed on the basis of knowledge, technical skills or professional behaviour demonstrated by the learner, depending on the focus of the clinical encounter. This should be followed by detailed feedback on the performance, self-reflection on how the learner performed and mutual development of plans for future learning and professional development.

In practice, there are potential problems inherent in both the assessments and the learning that arises from them (Schuwirth and van der Vleuten, 2006). The model of professional competence constructed by van der Vleuten (1996) makes clear that performance during assessment is affected by the type of task being assessed, a departure from the traditional trait view of competence, whereby generic knowledge and skills allow consistent performance across tasks. Under the new training regime, expertise involves development in knowledge and skills confined to specific areas and contexts that are acquired through experiences at work; they are not often generalisable across tasks or situations. This has implications for assessment, as what is measured at a test will depend on the learner's cognitive and reasoning processes; these will vary between individuals and also be different depending on learner experience and case complexity (van der Vleuten, 1996). Additionally, although assessment plays an important role in motivating learning (Crossley *et al.*, 2002), it may not facilitate retention of knowledge or its application to new situations; this may be because assessment methods often fail to provide a meaningful context and do not allow for repetition of performance, both of which are key to retention (Ericsson *et al.*, 1993).

Consequently, multiple assessments are required in different contexts in order to facilitate and measure the development of knowledge. The responsibility of providing these different contexts could well lie with the supervisors in their role of proving guided learning (Billett, 2001). Their active guidance would help learners appreciate the real benefit of assessment at work, which is to facilitate learning rather than just fulfilling mandatory requirements for training.

In response to the complexities involved in developing and assessing professional expertise, van der Vleuten (1996) suggests a simple framework for evaluating the utility of assessment methods. According to this framework, the usefulness of any assessment is determined by five variables: (1) reliability, (2) validity, (3) educational impact, (4) acceptability and (5) cost. These variables may carry different weight for different assessment methods, depending on the purpose of the assessment. This framework provides a theoretical basis for exploring the usefulness of assessment tools in practice because it takes into account not just the psychometric properties of the assessment methods, but also emphasises other aspects, such as end-user satisfaction and the feasibility of implementing these methods. In our research, we were interested in exploring the usefulness of the Royal College of Obstetricians and Gynaecologists' assessment methods, with an emphasis on the learning that was taking place alongside the assessment. Determining the reliability and validity of the assessment methods provides evidence of the psychometric rigour of the assessment; estimation of the cost of running the assessment provides us with an understanding of the practicalities of implementing such assessment in practice. However, the two variables that found synergy with Billett's framework of learning in the workplace were acceptability and educational impact, as both these variables would be affected positively if learners were satisfied that workplace assessment was enabling the development of expertise during their training. These two variables were studied in depth as proxy measures to understand how and to what extent learning may be occurring during assessment.

We employed a qualitative approach in our research and interviewed a purposive sample of 25 people involved in assessment within the specialty; this included both trainers and trainees. The interviews explored the views of participants on the acceptability and educational impact of the assessment, particularly focusing on how learning was thought to be facilitated during and as a result of assessment, with central reference to Billett's framework for guided learning.

Research findings

Billett developed his framework through research in a wide range of workplaces, including the social services, the manufacturing industry, hairdressing and coal mining. We applied Billett's notion of the development of expertise through learning at work and the progress from peripheral to full participation (Billett, 2001) as a basis for studying workplace assessment in medicine. We found that learning in the context of workplace assessment occurs as a result of guided learning (Billett, 2001) at the three levels described earlier, i.e. organising and managing learners' experiences in the workplace (first level), guidance in the development of procedures and understanding associated with work practice (second level) and development of self-regulated learning and ability to transfer knowledge and skills to other workplaces (third level).

Insights into the level and nature of such guided learning at work emerged from analysis of the interview data. There was some variation in the seniority of the trainers providing guidance during assessment. For the majority of assessment methods, senior assessors were found to be assessing most frequently, particularly in more complex cases. On the other hand, more junior grades of assessors were often asked to assess routine procedures, particularly outside standard working hours. From a learning perspective, it is reassuring that senior clinicians are providing expert supervision and assessment for most complex and non-routine procedures, fulfilling Billett's second-level guidance of 'modelling of tasks to be performed', demonstrating procedures to be learnt and 'making accessible knowledge that is hidden' (Billett, 2001, pp.142–3). For more routine procedures, less-experienced assessors may still qualify as experts as they become involved in more accountable tasks such as assessment while they progress from novice to expert during the course of their training. This is an area that is not well researched, with the majority of workplaces studied involving work that is almost always supervised by experts (Billett, 2001).

There was variation in uptake of the various types of assessments forms, with OSATS being much more likely to be completed than mini-CEX and CbD. This finding is similar to that reported elsewhere (Wilkinson *et al.*, 2008; Alves de Lima *et al.*, 2007) and reflects the extent to which organising workplace assessment in practice, i.e. the first level in Billett's model, is easy or difficult. Accordingly, skills that were less frequently seen in routine practice were obviously less likely to be supervised and assessed. OSATS were more likely to be completed as they frequently involve procedures that are normally supervised by seniors anyway and therefore do not require extra time commitment. For example, if an assessor is assisting a trainee during a caesarean section, it is easier for them to complete an OSATS at the end of the procedure:

> It is obstetrics and gynaecology – a practical subject, everybody wants to do the practical things with OSATS attached … the case-based discussions they can do when they've clerked somebody, and then they are presenting them, but then they have to tell the person initially that this is a case-based discussion

and there has got to be a little bit of time for discussion and for feedback. (Supervisor)

Arranging for supervision and assessment was sometimes quite difficult, especially outside normal working hours:

It is quite difficult to get consultants to come and assist you with caesarean sections and assist you with rotational deliveries or straightforward deliveries, because they just don't want to come and watch you do them. (Trainee)

In practice, and in keeping with Billett's first-level concept of 'organising and sequencing of workplace experience' (Billett, 2001, p.142), both supervisors and learners can select cases to be assessed on, attempting to sequence tasks 'which take the learner from being a novice to expert and from peripheral involvement to full participation in the workplace' (Billett, 2001, p.142). While learner-led selection of cases, and indeed assessors, may reflect their initiative in facilitating assessment, in the interview data, there was some concern that this would fail to provide a true reflection of an individual trainee's clinical performance and progress:

But you can also find if Mr X is an easy person … you will go and find him and make him fill that [form] and if Mr X is a difficult person, you will avoid him. Unless this is incorporated into a standard assessment, in every case, it won't work. (Supervisor)

This example highlights an important weakness in the way workplace assessment has been implemented in practice. Culturally, supervisors and learners often perceive assessment as a means to fulfil mandatory requirements that will allow trainees to progress in their training. The true educational impact of assessment facilitating learning and helping in the development of expertise is often undervalued. An appreciation of learning from assessment is one of the challenges faced by medical educators.

There are some recommendations on the optimal numbers of each type of form that trainees must complete each year. This means that trainees are assessed several times in different contexts, allowing supervisors to form a judgement on their competence in performing different tasks with different content (Eva et al., 1998). It also has the advantage of motivating trainees to complete their assessment, especially since they often only take seriously activities that they are assessed on (van der Vleuten, 1996). Multiple assessments provide multiple and repetitive learning stimuli that facilitate the development of professional knowledge (van der Vleuten, 1996) and expertise through deliberate practice (Ericsson *et al.*, 1993). On the other hand, once trainees realise that assessment provides little learning, they become less motivated to complete them, with resultant reduction in their educational impact (van der Vleuten *et al.*, 2010). Moreover, in dictating a fixed number of forms to be completed for the purpose of summative assessments, there is a tendency for both trainees and trainers to 'play the game', whereby trainees only complete the bare minimum of assessments (van der Vleuten *et al.*, 2010).

Our research findings suggest that there is a recognised need to promote a culture of learning from workplace assessment in medicine, both at organisation level (i.e. first level in Billett's model) and individual level (i.e. second level in Billett's model). This would involve emphasising that the purpose of workplace assessment is not only for assessing trainees but also, and more important, for facilitating learning, improving clinical and generic skills, and 'monitoring learners' progress and avoidance of learning inappropriate knowledge' (Billett, 2001, p.143). This was expressed through concerns that some trainers and trainees viewed these assessment forms simply as a tick-box exercise:

> Trainees often look at them [the forms] not as learning tools … they are looking at them as almost a kind of tick boxes at the end of their session when they feel they are capable of doing it [the procedure] … that's probably a cultural thing that will gradually change. (Supervisor)

One of the main objectives of workplace assessment is to provide formative guidance, via assessment, on how trainees are performing relative to standards expected for their stage of training. This guidance is in keeping with the third level of Billett's concept of guided learning, which requires supervisors to 'encourage the comparison of individual's progress with that of others' (Billett, 2001, p.143). This guidance may come from discussion and/or feedback that occurs either during the performance of the procedure itself (e.g. during a surgical case) or, as is more usual, following the performance alongside completion of the assessment forms (Norcini and Burch, 2007). Learning from feedback is recognised as key for the development of professional skills (Kalusmeir and Goodwin, 1975) and most workplace assessment methods have incorporated feedback as part of the assessment process. The techniques for facilitating discussion and providing feedback both have underpinnings in the theories discussed. Supervisors often use questions to facilitate discussion and feedback, a strategy suggested by Billett, for example, starting by asking the trainee how they thought the performance went, why they did things in a particular way and whether they could have performed differently. This allows trainees to articulate reasons for their actions, especially if they have demonstrated adaptation techniques to deal with new or challenging situations or tasks (Piaget, 1966).

In our research, trainees indicated that the immediate feedback following assessment was useful for their learning and provided them with an opportunity to plan their learning requirements based on what was discussed following assessment. This finding resonates with perceived educational impact from van der Vleuten's framework:

> We learn from the [assessment] because of the feedback that you get. With the OSATS, I do learn from them because you get feedback on the technique that you've done ... if you've done a good job, you also get praise. And, because you do OSATS with different people, often during the feedback, you get little tricks from different senior colleagues so you can learn from them. (Trainee)

Supervisors also thought that these assessment tools allowed them to provide structured feedback to their trainees:

> I am pretty good at feedback ... but I'm not sure that all consultants are ... it gives consultants a structured format ... and saying 'You did that well ... and this needs work' ... then I think they are excellent. (Supervisor)

Both supervisors and trainees felt that they needed to be more proactive in using these assessments in a more formative manner, rather than leaving them till just prior to trainees' annual assessment. This reflects an important component of the first level of guided learning in Billett's framework, in that sequencing tasks and staggering feedback would allow learners to foster their learning as they made progress:

> [They have] lots of positive features if they are done properly, i.e. not 'I have to do 10 of these forms and now I have two weeks to do them' ... if they are done throughout the year, it actually gives the trainee and the trainer time together. (Supervisor)

The staggering of assessment and subsequent feedback also allows trainees to evaluate the evidence of their own progress and to 'understand the breadth of the applicability of what they have learned' (Billett, 2001, p.143), part of the third level of Billett's framework. However, some trainees who do not space their assessments miss out on this element of assessment guiding learning.

Workplace encounters are often used by learners as opportunities that allow them to be observed by and receive feedback from experts (Jensen *et al.*, 2009; Wiles *et al.*, 2007). In addition, there are reports of the benefit of trainees sharing clinical information with assessors during the assessment process, thereby enhancing their knowledge and skills (Holmboe *et al.*, 2004). There was discussion around this during the interviews:

> We do learn from them because of the feedback that you get at the time the form is done … I know from the CbDs it's great because it makes you go in-depth into the topic that is being discussed and you have the opportunity to ask questions about it and often when I have done CbDs, I am motivated to go read the topic following filling out the CbD. (Trainee)

Within the third level of Billetts' guided learning framework, 'engaging learners in opportunities to reflect on what they have learnt' is an integral element (Billett, 2001, p.143). The concept of maintenance of 'equilibrium' within the cognitive structure (Piaget, 1966) affords further dimension to the analysis here. This equilibrium is characterised by a cognitive structure that is stable despite adaptations and mental compensations in response to environmental changes. Disequilibrium that results as the individual matures and gains more experience causes equilibration to occur as part of increasing intellectual functioning. For example, a learner moving from less to more complex and accountable tasks will learn to readjust equilibrium to incorporate new knowledge or skills. Equilibration that occurs in specific learning situations is of particular interest to teachers. For example, if a learner is found to be underperforming in particular tasks, then this may be indicative of disequilibrium in practice. The trainer should be able to assess whether the learner is finding it difficult to maintain equilibrium when faced with a new or different task. An appreciation of this aspect of learning would enable learners to reflect more constructively on their performance and accept feedback from the assessors more positively. The application of equilibration is that teachers should try and present problems that are above the student's level – this will cause disequilibrium and the learner will try to equilibrate. At the same time, the problem should be within the limits of adaptation and learners should be asked to explain their reasoning as part of self-reflection and response to feedback.

Self-assessment of performance during workplace assessment is an important aspect of development of expertise (Stevenson, 1994) and part of the development of self-regulation within the third level of Billett's guided learning framework (Billett, 2001). In the context of workplace assessment in medicine, it is our experience that there are two levels at which reflection may take place: trainees may reflect on the performance itself or reflect on the discussion and feedback from their trainers. Reflection on performance usually occurs during feedback from the trainer, providing an opportunity for assisted reflection. Using questions such as those described earlier (Billett, 2001) helps engage trainees in immediate self-reflection on how the performance went. It also allows trainees to acknowledge reasons for disequilibrium in clinical situations that proves to be challenging and to identify strategies that they adopted to maintain equilibrium and complete the task satisfactorily. These strategies could then be drawn upon in future. This raises the issue of transferability of skills, a notion that is present in both van der Vleuten's and Billett's frameworks. Self-assessment allows trainees to think about which skills acquired could be transferred to different clinical contexts and situations, and which cannot (third level in Billett's framework). Generic surgical skills, e.g. handling tissues, may well be transferable to other surgical procedures. The lack of transferability of expertise across different skills, on the other hand, reflects the need to have different assessment methods to assess different areas of expertise. For example, assessment criteria for specific procedures may need to be different from those for assessment of communication skills or professionalism.

In our research, one consequence of reflection on the performance and feedback as a result of assessment was that the trainee decides whether or not to approach particular trainers for future assessment. This may be because the trainee feels that some trainers are particularly harsh; this is certainly an issue in medicine, where a large proportion of workplace assessment is trainee-led and self-selection of assessors based on previous experiences is often seen. This finding seems to run counter to Billett's framework, in which guided learning is a mutual responsibility of supervisors and learners, and further reiterates the point made earlier about the need to enhance a culture of workplace learning alongside assessment in medicine.

Conversely, trainees sometimes recognise the limited educational impact (van der Vleuten, 1996) of assessment by a supervisor who does not discriminate between a good and a poor performance:

> Sometimes you just get someone who will just tick all the way down in the excellent box and that's just completely useless because it's not helping me …

> I'd rather they told me where my problem is, so I can work on it rather than just ticking excellent because they think that's what I want to hear. (Trainee)

Another drawback of workplace assessment tools is that in an attempt to make them more objective, they sometimes have a tendency to become reductionist, a problem noted in other forms of assessment as well (Norman *et al.*, 1991). In our study, they were often criticised for oversimplifying complex clinical skills assessment and focusing on checklists rather than assessment of holistic learning. They were also perceived as only being useful for assessing skills to a minimum standard. For example, some of the assessors in our study thought that these methods could not necessarily distinguish between average and high-performing trainees, an integral component of the third level of Billett's guided learning framework. This could be demotivating to the higher achievers:

> It gives you a superficial kind of evidence … this person can do the job, but I don't think it differentiates between a person who can do the job and a person who is very good at the job. (Supervisor)

Some participants highlighted the pitfall of focusing mainly on ticking the boxes rather than judging the overall clinical performance based on trainee experience and expertise. This could be demoralising for trainees and not allow the engagement and encouragement of learners required as part of the third level of Billett's framework on guided learning:

> They are not fully reflective of my abilities generally because it may have been a very difficult caesarean section that I struggled with or it may have been a straightforward first caesarean … I don't feel that they distinguish between those two things. (Trainee)

Reflective practice through assessment was highlighted as being useful in having a positive educational impact on the quality of the clinical care provided subsequently. This reflected the notion of 'abstraction of learning from one situation to another' (Billett, 2001, p.143), part of the third level of Billett's framework:

> I think it improves patient care because on a number of occasions, we've been filling in the feedback form and that has sometimes prompted an action for patient care that otherwise wouldn't have happened … because we were discussing the case more fully other things came to light and different actions were taken based on the discussion. (Trainee)

This improvement provides some evidence of the perceived educational impact of assessment, part of van der Vleuten's framework, and, given the difficulty in measuring the real impact on patient care, is a useful proxy measure of effectiveness.

Conclusions

In this chapter, we set out how Billett's strategy for effective workplace learning can be used to explore how learning takes place alongside assessment in the context of medicine. In particular, Billett's concept of guided learning in the workplace, together with Piaget's theory of cognitive development, provides us with a theoretical lens to explore a largely under-researched area in education. It allows us to evaluate workplace assessment, not just as a means for assessing performances but also, and more important, as a vehicle for expert guidance, feedback and reflection on performance to facilitate learning. Identifying ways in which learning occurs during workplace assessment will influence curriculum development and the design and implementation of assessment methods, and perhaps significantly engage both learners and experts in collaborative learning and assessment.

The main strength of this approach, at least in the context of medicine, lies in making assessment more relevant, challenging the misconception that workplace assessment is a tick-box exercise that needs to be completed in order to progress in the profession. It promises a richer context for learning in the clinical workplace. However, there are challenges to this approach. One of these is the inherent difficulty in measuring the quality of learning that is taking place and the impact, if any, that this has on professional practice. What is easier to evaluate is the perception of people engaged in learning and assessment and the value that they place on the learning. In addition, simply theorising workplace assessment and learning will not solve the main barriers to learning from assessment, including cultural and organisational issues, personal biases against structured assessment and cost. In particular, there appears to be a pressing need to educate both supervisors and learners on the major developmental purpose of workplace assessment and how best to maximise the benefit of such assessments to enhance future learning and professional practice. Further research needs to build on results from studies adopting more generic theoretical perspectives to improve our understanding of learning and assessment in the workplace and to allow us to be more effective in facilitating the development of professional expertise. In particular, Billett's framework of guided learning provides a methodology for exploring the nature of learning in the context of assessment. Moreover, van der Vleuten's framework allows us to build on this exploration, to actually evaluate the quality and educational impact of this learning.

Acknowledgements

The Royal College of Obstetricians and Gynaecologists, UK, funded the research on work-based assessment reported upon in this chapter.

References

Alves de Lima, A., Barrero, C., Baratta, S., *et al*. (2007) Validity, reliability, feasibility and satisfaction of the Mini-Clinical Evaluation Exercise (Mini-CEX) for cardiology residency training. *Medical Teacher*, 29(8), 785–90.

Billett, S. (1993) What's in a setting? Learning in the workplace. *Journal of Adult and Community Education*, 33(1), 4–14.

Billett, S. (1996) Constructing vocational knowledge: history, communities and individuals. *Journal of Vocational Education*, 48(2), 141–54.

Billett, S. (1999) Guided learning at work. In: D. Boud and J. Garrick (eds) *Understanding Learning at Work*. London, Routledge, pp.151–64.

Billett, S. (2000) Guided learning at work. *Journal of Workplace Learning*, 12(7), 272–85.

Billett, S. (2001) *Learning in the Workplace: strategies for effective practice*. Sydney, Allen & Unwin.

Bybee, R. W. and Sund, R. B. (1982) *Piaget for Educators*. 2nd edn. Long Grove, IL, Waveland Press.

Crossley, J., Humphris, G. and Jolly, B. (2002) Assessing health professionals. *Medical Education*, 36(9), 800–4.

Elstein, A. S., Shulman, L. S. and Sprafka, S. A. (1978) *Medical Problem Solving: an analysis of clinical reasoning*. Cambridge, MA, Harvard University Press.

Ericsson, K. A., Krampe, R. T. and Tesch-romer, C. (1993) The role of deliberate practice in the acquisition of expert performance. *Psychological Review*, 100(3), 363–406.

Eva, K. W., Neville, A. J. and Norman, G. R. (1998) Exploring the etiology of content specificity: factors influencing analogic transfer and problem solving. *Academic Medicine*, 73(10 Suppl.), S1–5.

Garvey, B. (1994) 'Ancient Greece, MBAs, the health service and George'. *Education and Training*, 36(2), 18–24.

Gay, B. (1994) 'What is mentoring?' *Education and Training*, 36(5), 4–7.

Holmboe, E. S., Yepes, M., Williams, F., *et al*. (2004) Feedback and the mini clinical evaluation exercise. *Journal of General Internal Medicine*, 19(5 Pt. 2), 558–61.

Jensen, A. R., Wright, A. S, Calhoun, K. E., *et al*. (2009) Validity of the use of objective structured assessment of technical skills (OSATS) with videorecorded surgical task performance. *Journal of the American College of Surgeons*, 209(3), S110–11.

Kalusmeier, H. J. and Goodwin, W. (1975) *Learning and Human Abilities: education psychology.* 4th edn. New York, NY, Harper & Row.

Lave, J. (1990) The culture of acquisition and the practice of understanding. In: J. W. Stigler, R. A. Shweder and G. H. Herdt (eds) *Cultural Psychology: essays on comparative human development.* Cambridge, Cambridge University Press, pp.259–86.

Lave, J. and Wenger, E. (1991) *Situated Learning: legitimate peripheral participation.* Cambridge, Cambridge University Press.

Norcini, J. and Burch, V. (2007) Workplace-based assessment as an educational tool: AMEE Guide No. 31. *Medical Teacher*, 29(9), 855–71.

Norman, G. R., van der Vleuten, C. P. and De Graaff, E. (1991) Pitfalls in the pursuit of objectivity: issues of validity, efficiency and acceptability. *Medical Education*, 25(2), 119–26.

Piaget, J. (1966) *Psychology of Intelligence.* Totowa, NJ, Littlefield, Adam & Company.

Schuwirth, L. W. T. and van der Vleuten, C. P. M. (2006) Medical education: challenges for educationalists. *British Medical Journal*, 333(7567), 544–6.

Setna, Z., Jha, V., Boursicot, K. A., *et al.* (2010) Evaluating the utility of workplace based assessment tools for speciality training. *Best Practice and Research: Clinical Obstetrics and Gynaecology*, 24(6), 767–82.

Stevenson, J. C. (1994) *Cognition at Work: the development of vocational expertise.* Adelaide, National Centre for Vocational Education Research.

Temple, J. (2010) *Time for Training: a review of the impact of the European Working Time Directive on the quality of training.* Available from: www.mee.nhs.uk/pdf/JCEWTD_Final%20report.pdf (accessed 30 January 2012).

Van der Vleuten, C. P. M. (1996) The assessment of professional competence: developments, research and practical implications. *Advances in Health Sciences Education*, 1(1), 41–67.

Van der Vleuten, C. P. M., Schuwirth, L. W., Scheele, F., *et al.* (2010) The assessment of professional competence: building blocks for theory development. *Best Practice and Research: Clinical Obstetrics and Gynaecology*, 24(6), 703–19.

Wiles, C. M., Dawson, K., Hughes, T. A., *et al.* (2007) Clinical skills evaluation of trainees in a neurology department. *Clinical Medicine*, 7(4), 365–9.

Wilkinson, J. R., Crossley, J. G, Wragg, A., *et al.* (2008) Implementing workplace-based assessment across the medical specialties in the United Kingdom. *Medical Education*, 42(4), 364–73.

4

Developing a social constructivist model of nursing's pedagogic practice using Bernstein's educational theories

Stephen O'Connor

Introduction: social constructivism and the analysis of pedagogic discourse

In this chapter I will describe how sociological theory was used to analyse the assumptions that underpin the field of nurse education. This is by means of 'extended philosophical analysis' (Harré and Secord, 1972) of the discipline's public forms of thought as represented by a sample of its published literature or 'pedagogic discourse', defined for the purposes of this work as any written artefact that represents 'the field talking about itself' (Maton, 2004, p.61). Dowling (1999) argues that within this context, 'the reading of texts becomes a research activity to the extent that it enables or proceeds from a theorising of the activity to which the text is to be referred' (accessed 13/2/2011). This means that the selection, analysis and reporting of texts describing a particular phenomenon are guided by one or more theoretical frameworks or 'refractory prisms' (Maton, 2004) that provide a symbolic depiction of those phenomena. The theories themselves can also be subjected to confirmation or disconfirmation however, on the basis of their ability to accurately predict, describe, explain or prescribe responses to those phenomena (Chinn and Kramer, 1991) in a 'continuous movement between theory and data' (Maton, 2004, p.72).

The purpose of extended philosophical analysis is twofold: first, to identify hidden patterns, contradictions or assumptions present within a particular phenomenon (in this case, the knowledges, texts or discourses of nurse education) from the perspective of the theoretical framework, and second, to subject that framework to confirmation or disconfirmation on the basis of its ability to predict, describe, explain or prescribe what might be found within that narrative. The 'theorising on theory' that follows the production of the narrative has been described as 'discursive fieldwork' by Bernstein (2000, p.xvi), but within Bernsteinian theory, the theory tested in such a way should provide adequate description of its underlying concepts, principles and assumptions to make this possible. It should, therefore, provide a robust and comprehensive explanation of the phenomenon and not be dependent on other theories to make sense of it. In Bernstein's words, it should 'posit an explication of the inner logic of pedagogic discourse and its practices … the rules of its construction, circulation, contextualisation, acquisition and change' (1996, p.4). By this, Bernstein means that educational theory should not only explain what kind of learning takes place but also why (i.e. its inner logic) and how (i.e. its practices). This occurs through an explication of the ways in which different kinds of knowledge are discovered or constructed by researchers, practitioners or theorists; validated, hierarchically organised and circulated within formal or informal curricula by experts in the field; contextualised or recontextualised by those responsible for teaching that knowledge; and acquired or adapted to the situational contingencies of patient care by those working in clinical practice. As such, it represents an all-encompassing, or 'meta-theory', of educational discourse.

In this chapter, I will illustrate how theory developed by the late British educational sociologist Basil Bernstein was used to analyse the pedagogic discourse of nurse educators and others in formal positions of power within the field of nurse education, and identify how reified practices and habituations within the field are socially and culturally constructed (Buckley, 2004). In this respect, the work is unashamedly social constructivist in nature; that is, it holds to the view that meaning, learning and knowledge are created by means of social interaction, as individuals observe, share, discuss and debate different ideas, experiences and perspectives about a particular phenomenon. Shotter (1993) supports this view, arguing that meaning and sense making are primarily 'conversational or responsively relational' (p.161), which means that they occur through a series of complex social relations in which each and every interaction is perceived, analysed and acted upon differently by each social actor involved in the interaction.

It has been hypothesised that the social relations of pedagogic activity within nursing would be discernible through a 'close reading of the text' (Rolfe and Freshwater, 2005, p.368) contained within the discourse, since this represents a conversation between different individuals or groups as part of a transmitter–acquirer relationship. Buckley (2004) argues that in so doing, it is possible to 'deliver accurate information about the ways in which we attribute our intuitions [about practice]' (p.7) within any social field. Moreover, a social constructivist stance is appropriate since it is 'principally concerned with elucidating the processes by which people come to describe, explain or otherwise account for the world in which they live' (Gergen, 1985, pp.3–4), and provides a useful tool by which our own social practices as teachers, researchers and clinicians can be analysed and held up to the scrutiny of others (Reay, 2004).

Harré and Secord (1972) argue that 'conversation [should] be thought of as creating a social world just as causality generates a physical one' (p.65), and Bernstein himself asserted that pedagogic discourse 'can describe something other than itself' (Bernstein, 1996, p.136), primarily as a result of 'recontextualisation', the process by which conversation, dialogue or discourse is transformed into something other than the sum of its parts. For Bernstein, recontextualisation is the primary function of the teacher, who is concerned with taking others' oftentimes complex ideas (or discourses) and placing them within a more general narrative that can be better understood by others. From a social constructivist perspective, however, it is acknowledged that the very act of recontextualising others' work into a more readily understandable narrative 'often decides how a particular theory is to be positioned' (Bernstein, 2000, p.xvi). This means that the act of recontextualisation changes the nature and emphasis of the theory in relation to the context in which the teaching takes place and those other theories alongside which it is taught. Bernstein's work has been considered particularly useful for this purpose since his theories provide perhaps, the most comprehensive explanation of the ways in which pedagogic discourse can be used to 'regulate the relationships between power, social groups, forms of consciousness and forms of practice' (Bernstein, 1996, p.28). That is to say, his theories can explain how teachers' attributions about the production, legitimation and dissemination of knowledge claims have the effect of shaping the application of that knowledge and overcome the suggestion that (nurse) pedagogy has no voice of its own in the often heated debate about the theory–practice gap (Bernstein, 2000; Rafferty et al., 1996).

However, before discussing the contribution that Bernstein's theory is capable of making to the field of nurse education, it is first necessary to describe the broad sweep or 'conceptual architecture' of a life's work that spanned many decades and included both empirical and theoretical analysis of some of the most important sociological themes influencing education during the course of the twentieth century. In the next section, I will therefore provide a brief overview of relevant Bernsteinian theories, including his writings on visible and invisible curricula, the 'classification' and 'framing' of professional knowledge, and vertical and horizontal knowledge structures. These theories demonstrate how pedagogic discourses are regulated by those holding symbolic or actual power over the pedagogic activities of the field by means of the 'pedagogic device', the rules by which knowledges, texts and discourses are reproduced in the practice domain through the pedagogic agency of teachers. This will provide the basis for the last section in this chapter, in which I specifically address his notion of 'pedagogic discourse' and introduce my own conceptualisation of pedagogic practice based on Bernstein's theories. This model will then be used to explain how those engaged in nurse education unwittingly make use of complex distribution, recontextualisation and evaluation rules drawn from his theories when assembling knowledges, texts and discourses from the field of knowledge production into visible pedagogies or curricula 'for the purposes of their selective transmission and acquisition' (Bernstein, 1974) in the practice setting.

Tracing the development of Bernstein's theory and its possible contribution to nurse education

In an obituary written shortly after Bernstein's death in September 2000, Davies (2001) wrote that Bernstein was 'the most interesting and the most important British sociologist of recent times, internationally better known for longer than any other' and responsible for providing 'the most developed grammar for under-standing the shape and character of our current educational practice' (p.1). Ever responsive to social change and a prolific commentator on educational issues, Bernstein's published works reflect not only the genesis of his own ideas but also mirror the evolution of educational sociology itself, starting with his early interest in social class and sociolinguistic theory in the 1950s and 1960s, and hence to his growing interest in visible and invisible pedagogies and the classification and framing of educational knowledge in the 1970s. By the following decade, he had moved on to consider the structuring of pedagogic discourse itself, and from there, to analyse how knowledge structures are themselves generated. This last phase of his work existed only in a nascent form at the time of his death, but has since been expanded upon by others (Moore, 2006; Arnot and Reay, 2004; Gamble, 2004; Hasan, 2004; Muller, 2004). Bernstein's works provide a useful theoretical prism therefore, through which almost every aspect of pedagogic practice can be analysed, and which can also be used to explain the role played by teachers in the social replication of nursing knowledge. To date, only a few authors have attempted to apply his works to nursing – namely, Thomas and Davies (2006), O'Connor (2007) and McNamara (McNamara *et al.*, 2011; McNamara, 2008). In order to address this omission, I will now consider how the canon of professional knowledge (for any field) is collected, codified and legitimised within an explicit, visible curriculum through the refractory prism of Bernstein's theories before discussing further their implications for nurse education.

Visible and invisible curricula and the classification and framing of professional knowledge

Bernstein first introduced his ideas on the classification and framing of educational knowledge in his contribution to Michael Young's book *Knowledge and Control: new directions for the sociology of education* (Bernstein, 1971b). The chapter also included his ideas on 'collection' and 'integrated' curriculum codes. The former are characterised by strongly boundaried knowledge areas or 'subject singulars' (such as mathematics or physics) which are autonomous of developments in other subjects or disciplinary fields, in contrast to the latter, which are more loosely defined, less autonomous, and which draw heavily upon the curricula or knowledge bases of other fields or disciplines, as nursing invariably does (Walford, 1995). As vehicles for the production, reproduction and distribution of professional knowledge, Bernstein suggested that a field or discipline's professional curriculum reflects the outcome of differential power relations both within the field, and between those closely associated with it (e.g. medicine, nursing, social work, physiotherapy). Hence, those disciplines with longer established and more distinct identities or knowledge bases, such as law or medicine, have more strongly classified curricula than neophyte professions or those with less distinct knowledge bases, such as nursing. Thus, while the core concepts, competencies and knowledges required to practice medicine are well codified within a clearly integrated visible curricula with a vertical knowledge structure (*see* the next section), and there is clear signification between the importance of different kinds of knowledge and a linear logic to their delivery, there is far greater uncertainty about what should be included in the visible curriculum of nurse education programmes, how this should be ordered, and where it should come from. The papers by Aranda and Law (2007) and McPherson (2008) on the role of sociology within the nursing curriculum are but two examples of the continuing debate about what constitutes legitimate nursing knowledge, arguments about sociology's role within the curriculum going back many years to a sometimes vitriolic debate between Porter (1995) and Sharp (1995, 1994) over the issue.

No wonder then, that those responsible for developing nursing curricula often display 'considerable uncertainty … about what forms of knowledge should be taught' (Christie, 2007, p.8), most relying instead upon the 'mandatory curriculum enforced by a detailed syllabus and list of learning requirements' handed down by the various professional bodies governing nurse registration in a devolved United Kingdom (Thomas and Davies, 2006, p.573). These sometimes appear to have been influenced by those taking an anti-academic stance towards the education of nurses (Meirs, 2002; Bradshaw, 2001), and yet Bernstein considered professional knowledge to be 'uncommonsense knowledge', which is freed from the particular, the mundane or the specific through forms of language and inquiry that 'make possible either the creation or the discovery of new realities' (Bernstein, 2003 p.99). There is, interestingly, a clear relationship between the higher-order thinking suggested by Bernstein's theories about professional knowledge and the much-vaunted ambition of nurse education programmes to create reflective practitioners who are critical in their thinking and professional in their actions, although the extent to which this can be achieved in a culture which values doing rather than thinking, compliance rather than critical inquiry and competence rather than performance is questionable (Cowan *et al.*, 2007, 2005; Norman *et al.*, 2002; Sabin, 2001). Furthermore, the subordination of nursing's 'subject singular' (i.e. the knowledge, texts and discourses comprising nursing's unique knowledge base) to the requirements of interprofessional learning (Walsh *et al.*, 2005; Glen, 2004; Camsookai, 2002) are but two examples of the way in which a lack of balance in power relations between nurse educators and those exerting external control over the health education agenda (i.e. politicians, managers, policymakers and so forth) are irrevocably shaping nurse education.

Summarising the concepts of classification and framing for the purposes of this chapter therefore, it is sufficient to state that classification refers to the degree to which a specific profession, field or academic discipline is insulated from the influence or control of these external influences so that its members enjoy a high degree of professional autonomy. Developing a distinctive knowledge base and maintaining a high level of control over the production and social reproduction of that knowledge base through a clearly articulated curriculum, selective entry to the field of study, and an accentuated sense of professional habitus are how this is achieved (O'Connor, 2007). Thus, strongly classified subjects, fields or disciplines have their own knowledges, texts and discourses which are separate and distinct from those of their comparators. In contrast, weakly classified fields are, in part at least, reliant upon the knowledges, texts and discourses of other disciplines or subject fields, and have porous curricula which are often horizontally and segmentally organised, the significance of which I will now discuss in relation to nurse education.

Vertical and horizontal knowledge structures and their significance for nurse education

Bernstein defined hierarchical knowledge structures as those which:
- have coherent, explicit and systematically principled structures
- are hierarchically organised
- attempt to create very general propositions and theories that integrate knowledge at lower levels
- consequently show underlying uniformities across an expanding range of apparently different phenomena.

Within vertical knowledge structures, there are 'strong distributive rules regulating access, transmission and evaluation' (Bernstein, 1999, p.157), the development of the curriculum being accomplished through a series of tacit rules or 'distributive procedures' (p.157) which govern the selection, evaluation, legitimisation and codification of knowledges into a hierarchically organised knowledge base. One good example of this is medicine, in which the study of pathology is predicated upon the student having first acquired knowledge of anatomy and physiology, and the prescribing of medicines is dependent upon their first having studied the field of pharmacology, and so forth. The relationship between different knowledges is linear, so that the development of competence or professional performance in one area is dependent upon the student gaining proficiency in the knowledges considered foundational for their performance at an every higher level of complexity. In contrast to this, the relationship between knowledges contained within an horizontal knowledge structure can only be assumed (Moore, 2006), Bernstein arguing that, 'the segmental organisation of knowledges of horizontal discourse leads to segmentally structured acquisitions [since] there is no necessary relations between what is learned in different segments' (1996, p.159). Therefore, in comparison with vertical knowledge structures, which are linear, incremental and highly regulated, horizontal knowledge structures draw upon the knowledges of many disciplines, and their relevance to the discipline in question may only become apparent when directed 'towards specific, immediate goals highly relevant to the acquirer in the context of his or her life' (p.159).

Thus, the immediate relevance of sociology, social policy or even, perhaps, psychology, will not immediately seem relevant to the neophyte student of nursing who regards these 'non-nursing' knowledges as superfluous to the nurse's role as a 'carer'. As a consequence, their importance only becomes apparent when arranging the discharge of a patient with complex social, psychological and, perhaps, financial difficulties into the community. Segmental learning within a horizontal knowledge structure is dependent therefore, upon situational context, and the practitioner needs to draw upon a repertoire of knowledge, the relevance of which may not have been apparent at the time of its acquisition. Within this context, the strength of the social base or interaction between members of the field in specific clinical settings is also highly important, since pedagogic activity in a horizontally organised knowledge structure relies to a great extent upon social 'exchange' than on the 'distribution' or 'circulation' of formal learning from a hierarchically delineated curriculum or knowledge base. This explains, too, the important role of clinical mentors, academic tutors or preceptors in helping neophyte practitioners to make these connections through reflection and discussion of case exemplars drawn from practice.

Bernstein (1996) argues that learning in this instance 'is likely to be oral, local … multi-layered, and contradictory across, but not within cases' (p.157), so that the learner acquires a repertoire of 'schemas' or case exemplars which may or may not be usefully applied to other patients or settings. Crucially, however, there may still appear to be little connection between theory and practice where learning occurs in such a way, and the linkages between the two are more tacit than explicit in nature. Similarly, knowledges, skills and competencies acquired in one work-based learning environment may seem equally ephemeral in another, and have to be adapted or unlearnt completely in the next as students struggle to relate the outputs of prior learning to a new and often very different clinical environment. In such circumstances, 'there is no necessary relation between what is learned in the different segments … they are contextually specific and context dependent, embedded in on-going practices, usually with strong affective loading, and are directed at specific, immediate goals' (Bernstein, 2000, p.159). The socially situated nature of this learning highlights the importance of social constructivist theory within nurse education, since 'social constructivism is principally concerned with elucidating the processes by which people come to describe, explain or otherwise account for the world in which they live' (Gergen,

1985, pp.3–4). This only explains half of the equation in respect of nurse education, however, since there is clearly a more explicit curriculum (or more correctly, a multitude of similar but distinct curricula) which govern the social reproduction of nursing, and it is to this more formal aspect of nurse education, and specifically the way that this is constructed and structured, that I will now turn my attention.

The structuring of pedagogic discourse

Bernstein (1981) suggests that pedagogic discourse 'arises out of the action of a group of specialised agents operating in a specialised setting in terms of the interests, often competing interests, in this setting' (p.327), an explanation that is well illustrated by the ethnographic study by Thomas and Davies (2006) of 25 nurse lecturers' knowledge of and participation in curriculum planning. In this, they identified one group of teachers who had more knowledge and experience of developing curricula than the others. These were fully conversant with the *specialised* languages associated with this activity – namely, the 'rules' underpinning curriculum development – and this enabled them to present their ideas to others in a more influential manner. Bernstein suggests that proficiency in the use of these specialised languages depends upon the accumulation of both the 'recognition rules' and the 'realisation rules' that govern pedagogic practice. Recognition rules govern the way in which social actors recognise the significance of the context in which they find themselves, while realisation rules describe how they subsequently produce texts or discourses relevant to that context (Morais and Neves, 2001, p.195). Thus, in Thomas and Davies's study there were different power relations between those familiar with the purpose and 'jargon' associated with curriculum development, and those unable to communicate their own ideas or preferences within that highly specialised context. Their study provides a good example of the way in which specific 'signification codes' (knowledges, texts and discourses) are used by a cadre of elite social actors within the field of education to appropriate the discourses of the field with the intention of 'bringing them into a special relation with each other for the purposes of their selective transmission and acquisition' (Bernstein, 2000, pp.183–4). Apple (1995) reiterates this:

> Although there is no formal right for everyone to be represented in debates over whose cultural capital, whose knowledge will be declared legitimate for transmission to future generations of students, it is still the case that a selective tradition operates in which only specific groups' knowledge becomes official knowledge. Thus, the freedom to help select the formal corpus of knowledge is bounded by power relations that have very real effects. (p.54)

As such, the knowledges, texts and discourses selected in this way become compromised by the very act of 'selection, simplification, condensation or elaboration' (Bernstein, 1986, p.227) by powerful 'recontextualising agents' so that the curriculum reflects their own interests and interpretations of the knowledges, texts and discourses of the field rather than those of people lacking the same degree of cultural fluency (Bernstein, 1986). Rafferty *et al.* (1996) describe these signification codes as 'epistemologies of esteem' and argues that these are used to legitimise the claims to expertise made by these individuals. The original object(s) of the curriculum and the 'grammar' used to describe it are subsequently recontextualised to take account of their own particular interests. Thus I have myself worked in a range of institutions which variously proclaimed their curricula to be 'patient centred', 'skills based' or 'problem based', and demonstrated completely different emphases in balance among the biomedical, social and 'nursing' sciences depending upon the prevailing zeitgeist or pedagogic biases of their originators.

Using the example of physics, Bernstein suggests that the logic of the teaching of physics cannot formally be derived from the logic of the science itself. Thus, there is scope for those holding an 'authorising skeptron' over the pedagogic activity of the field (Dowling, 2001) to dictate not only the content of the curriculum but also the way in which this is taught (Bernstein, 2000). Taken together, the recognition and realisation rules form the 'pedagogic device', the mechanism by which the pedagogic activity of a field (in terms of both its content and its delivery) is actualised. Control of the pedagogic device (Bernstein, 1990) enables a small group of practitioners within the field to regulate its pedagogic discourse in such a way that 'the dominant, higher status code modality of the field favours their own' (Maton, 2004, p.50). However, the way in which they do this, and the legitimations used to justify such claims, invariably bring one to the subject of how certain pedagogic discourses derive their importance, how they are structured, and how they are communicated in order to achieve the desired effect. I shall now discuss these within the context of a new conceptualisation of nurse education, one based upon Bernstein's theories and my own review of nursing's pedagogic discourse, although I am unable within this chapter to go into great detail about the discourses themselves.

Developing a Bernsteinian model of nurse pedagogy

I started this chapter with the hypothesis that Bernstein's work articulates a well-defined conceptualisation of pedagogic discourse capable of offering fresh insight into the practice of nurse education, but also lends itself to the possibility of verification through analysis of a sample of nursing's pedagogic discourse. In this respect, I found that his concepts were indeed relevant. I also found that his theories, which, for the most part, were developed within the context of compulsory (i.e. school) education, had relevance when transferred to an analysis of the higher education of nurses. In doing so, I also became aware of the importance of nurse educators creating space for themselves to develop their own pedagogic knowledges and recognising the primacy of this activity in their daily lives, rather than apologising for being neither wholly engaged in the field of research (knowledge production) or clinical practice (the field of reproduction). Instead, they needed to establish a unique place for themselves between these two domains. Fisher (2005), too, argues that nurse educators should place more emphasis on the need to become skilled educators than on unreasonable expectations that they also be expert clinicians, managers and researchers. Indeed, the noted educationalist Ramsden (1992) has pointed out that 'the professional authority of the academic-as-scholar rests on a body of knowledge', but in the same way, 'the professional authority of the academic-as-teacher should rest upon a body of didactic knowledge comprising knowledge of how the subject he or she professes is best learned and taught' (p.9), and it is this premise which guided the work thus described. This process is more advanced in some countries than others, but it is my contention that professionals must have strong conceptual models on which to base their practice. To this end, I have tentatively proposed a model of nurse education based upon Bernstein's theories (*see* Figure 4.1).

This model places the dominant discourses of those involved in the production, evaluation and validation of the field's knowledge base (such as researchers and, to a certain extent, opinion leaders) within the central or 'theoretical' domain. This indicates that, for the most part, they represent a small though significant subsection of the field of nursing that is primarily concerned with the production of nursing's propositional discourses and knowledge structures through research or the formulation of nurse education policy. These individuals consciously or unconsciously use the distribution rules of the field to frame a canon of literature and reify some discourses over others to create dominant, higher-status code modalities (i.e. the knowledge base) which those working

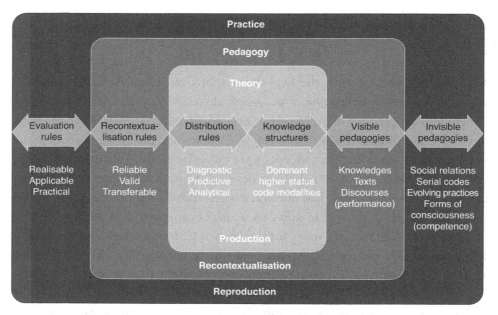

FIGURE 4.1 A Bernsteinian conceptualisation of nursing's pedagogic device

within the recontextualising domain (such as lecturers, teachers and practice educators) must first appropriate in order to bring them 'into a special relationship with each other for the purposes of their selective transmission and acquisition' (Bernstein, 1990, p.183–4). Within this context, those engaged in teaching are engaged to a greater or lesser extent in determining which of the prescribed knowledges are to be taught within nursing's visible pedagogy or curriculum; also, they determine when, where, how and in what order these are to be taught, through the recontextualising rules of the pedagogic device which determines both what is to be taught or reproduced within clinical practice and how this is to take place.

Within this domain, the espoused knowledges of the profession are rendered into more readily accessible learning activities through the recontextualising activities of the nurse educators. Their primary concern in relation to these is 'performativity' – that is, the ability of the students to demonstrate attainment of demonstrable learning outcomes that, it is hoped, are reliable, valid and transferable to the clinical setting or practice domain. These criteria are used to determine which of the knowledges legitimised by those in the field of production can successfully be reproduced as a result of pedagogic activity, bearing in mind the complex social relations, role identities, varying experiences and forms of consciousness affecting those in the field of practice. The role of the educator within the field of recontextualisation, therefore, is to act as a cultural arbiter between the reified knowledges, texts and discourses of those working in the field of knowledge production (theory) and the expectations, needs and 'profane' or practice-based knowledges of those engaged in the field of reproduction (practice), which Bernstein describes as being 'two faces of the same coin' (2000, p.54).

However, recontextualisation occurs at several levels of pedagogic activity. It may occur at the level of the entire field, exemplified by the authors of nursing textbooks, and by those writing national standards, guidelines, formulating national curricula or educational policies. It may also occur at the organisational level, where another group of educators are involved in the recontextualisation of those standards, national policies, curricula or guidelines, or the selection of published texts, knowledges and discourses, when developing curricula for their institutions (Thomas and Davies, 2006). Finally, it also occurs at the micro or classroom level, where the knowledges, texts and discourses prescribed by these curricula are again recontextualised within the teaching interaction to meet situational demands or the specific needs of individual students or groups.

Student performance is crucially important at this level, since this is also used to evaluate the performance of the teacher. As a consequence, the teacher 'places the emphasis upon a specific output of the acquirer, upon a particular text the acquirer is expected to construct, and upon the specialised skills necessary to the production of this specific output' (Bernstein, 2000, p.44) since performance measures will be used to judge students' fitness to practise and subsequently enter the professional register.

Having been recontextualised within what I have called the pedagogic domain, these knowledges, texts and discourses are then enacted within the field of reproduction (or practice domain) in order to shape the social relations, forms of consciousness and evolving practices of the field of nursing. Thus, students entering the field of practice are expected to be 'knowledgeable doers', and to make explicit use of the knowledge and skills they have learnt in the formal learning environment, even if the use of these skills may only be implicit to the observer. Thus, students who have fully assimilated the nursing values of 'patient-centred care' will behave in a 'patient-centred way' in practice. Moreover, in doing so, they may also draw upon other aspects of the horizontal knowledge structure of nursing, including psychological, sociological and social policy theory when, for example, managing the complex discharge previously mentioned or caring for a dying patient and family members. The explicit use of these knowledges cannot be controlled by those in the field of knowledge production, or, indeed, the field of recontextualisation, but are nevertheless applied selectively and with recourse to the situated contingencies encountered by the practitioner in the clinical setting.

However, when practising in a 'patient-centred' manner, it is important to note that practitioners are also developing their own highly situated and context-dependent series of case exemplars (or code modalities) in reaction to their experiences and those of their colleagues. These comprise the bulk of the discipline's invisible pedagogy, which is concerned primarily with the reproduction of social relations, forms of consciousness, role identity and professional habitus rather than reified knowledge structures; that is, what it 'means' to be a nurse and how a nurse should 'behave' rather than what they should 'know' (O'Connor, 2007). The overriding criteria for the development and use of these situated knowledges is not that they are reliable, valid or transferable, since the practitioners are not concerned with anything but the specifics of the situation in which they and their colleagues find themselves at that time. Indeed, the experiential knowledge gained in that situation may run counter to the knowledges conveyed within the formal or visible curriculum. Thus, a nurse who knows full well the dangers of smoking, but who wishes to practise in a 'patient-centred' manner, may turn a blind eye to this behaviour in a patient who is extremely anxious or disturbed, realising that this is likely to be the most effective palliative intervention for someone in a stressful situation and for whom it is a deeply engrained coping mechanism. The application of this particular, situated knowledge (i.e. knowledge of the patient and his or her overall condition) may supersede previously reified discourses about health promotion within the context of acting as a patient-centred carer in that instance.

Different pedagogic discourses are continuously being produced in each of the three domains within the model, but in each case the main difference is, 'the character of the knowledge that they produce and what counts as legitimate issues, questions, modes of inquiry and answers' (Moore, 2006, p.29). As a consequence, pedagogy from one level to the next is the process whereby 'somebody acquires new forms or develops existing forms of conduct, knowledge, practice and criteria from somebody or something deemed to be an appropriate provider and evaluator' (Bernstein, 1999, p.259), whether a university professor or reader, in relation to the findings of empirical research, a lecturer or senior lecturer in relation to propositional knowledge within the visible curriculum, or a clinical mentor or role model in relation to the invisible curriculum or social relations of the practice domain. One other feature of the model is that it places the pedagogic activity of those working within the recontextualising field as teachers or educators between the fields of knowledge production and reproduction, as

Bernstein's theory implies that it should. This acknowledges that those working within the pedagogic domain are uniquely placed to bridge the supposed theory–practice gap and make a 'conscious effort to clarify and define rules which are direct abstractions of situations in the clinical domain … abstractions [which often] have little meaning' (Landers, 2000 p.1550) in the clinical setting.

Concluding remarks

Nurse educators straddle a binary educational system that reifies propositional knowledge within a visible pedagogy that places emphasis upon the accumulation of socially constructed 'serial codes' (Bernstein, 1990, p.180) and an invisible pedagogy enacted within a practice environment over which they have little or no control. However, to date, most research within the field of nurse education has focused on the 'analysis of what is to be produced in and by education', rather than 'an analysis of the medium of reproduction' (Bernstein, 1999, p.166) – that is, the ways in which learning and the content of learning are socially constructed. However, Bernstein (1990) argues that 'any theory of education should have a theory of the pedagogic device', and suggests that 'such a theory could well be its necessary foundation and provide the theoretical object of the discipline' (p.190). This advice seems particularly salient as nurse educators prepare for the advent of an all-graduate profession. Moreover, it has been suggested that many regard nurse educators as little more than 'dabblers' in the field of knowledge production (Nolan *et al.*, 2008; Johnson, 2004; Hill *et al.*, 2003), and the compulsion 'to produce empirically driven studies rather than papers that are conceptual or theoretical in nature' (Haigh, 2005, p.342) means that the study of nursing pedagogy has been eclipsed by the need to produce clinical research outputs in order to develop the research base of the profession. However, this has placed nurse education in the invidious position of constantly being on the back foot and susceptible to the transient whims of those dictating health and educational policy elsewhere. Thus, while the knowledge base of nursing has inevitably developed, there is little indication that this has been codified into a single, choate and hierarchically organised body of knowledge, at least in the United Kingdom, where teaching and educational research continue to be regarded as inferior activities in comparison with clinical research, or, indeed, clinical practice.

Current research-funding models actively dissuade both theoretical and pedagogic research projects (Parse, 2008, 1998), and this has resulted in a wide range of courses that differ hugely, in terms both of their content and of their delivery. Ironically, the few features that many different nursing curricula do have in common reflect the need to implement externally imposed clinical practice and competence requirements that are more redolent of an apprenticeship training model than a professional education, and this has undoubtedly affected our confidence as educators (Brennan, 2007; Beijaard *et al.*, 2004). It is appropriate and timely, therefore, to posit a new model of nursing pedagogy that makes explicit the equal and unique contribution made by those engaged in the field of knowledge production, recontextualisation and reproduction, as defined by the theories of Basil Bernstein. It is gratifying that Bernstein's theories seem to have a high 'truth value' (Sandelowski, 1986), and I hope that the model presented here will encourage nurse educators to develop a broader conceptualisation of the importance of their pedagogic activity and a stronger sense of habitus as teachers and nurse academics (O'Connor, 2007).

References

Apple, M. (1995) Official knowledge and the growth of the activist state. In: P. Atkinson, B. Davies, S. Delamont, *et al.* (eds) *Discourse and Reproduction: essays in honor of Basil Bernstein*. Cresskill, NJ, Hampton, pp.51–84.

Aranda, K. and Law, K. (2007) Tales of sociology and the nursing curriculum: revisiting the debates. *Nurse Education Today*, 27(6), 561–7.

Arnot, M. and Reay, D. (2004) The framing of pedagogic encounters: regulating the social order in classroom teaching. In: J. Muller, B. Davies and A. Morais (eds) *Reading Bernstein, Researching Bernstein*. London, RoutledgeFalmer, pp.135–51.

Beijaard, D., Meijer, P. C., and Verloop, N. (2004) Reconsidering research on teachers' professional identity. *Teacher and Teacher Education*, 20(2), 107–28.

Bernstein, B. (1971a) *Class, Codes and Control, Volume 1: theoretical studies towards a sociology of language*. London, Routledge & Kegan Paul.

Bernstein, B. (1971b) On the classification and framing of educational knowledge. In: M. F. D. Young (ed.) *Knowledge and Control: new directions for the sociology of education*. London, Collier-Macmillan, pp.47–69.

Bernstein, B. (1974) *Class, Codes and Control, Volume 1*. 2nd edn. London, Routledge & Kegan Paul.

Bernstein, B. (1981) Codes, modalities and the process of cultural reproduction: a model. *Language and Society*, 10(3), 327–63.

Bernstein, B. (1986) On pedagogic discourse. In: J. Richardson (ed.) *Handbook of Theory and Research in the Sociology of Education*. New York, Greenwood Press, pp.205–40.

Bernstein, B. (1990) *Class, Codes and Control, Volume 4: the structuring of pedagogic discourse*. London, Routledge & Kegan Paul.

Bernstein, B. (1996) *Pedagogy, Symbolic Control and Identity: theory, research, critique.* 1st edn. Lanham, MD, Rowman & Littlefield.

Bernstein, B. (1999) Vertical and horizontal discourse: an essay. *British Journal of Sociology of Education*, 20(2), 158–73.

Bernstein, B. (2000) *Pedagogy, Symbolic Control and Identity: theory, research and critique.* 2nd edn. Lanham, MD, Rowman & Littlefield.

Bernstein, B. (2003) *Class, Codes and Control. Volume III*. London, Routledge.

Bradshaw, A. (2001) *The Nurse Apprentice*. Aldershot, Ashgate.

Brennan, J. (2007) On researching ourselves: the difficult case of autonomy in researching higher education. *International Perspectives on Higher Education*, 4, 167–81.

Buckley, A. (2004) Social externalism, Segal and contradictory intuitions. Presented at the Warwick Graduate Conference on the Philosophy of the Mind, Warwick University, 27–28 November.

Camsookai, J. (2002) The role of the lecturer practitioner in interprofessional education. *Nurse Education Today*, 22(6), 466–75.

Chinn, P. L. and Kramer, M. K. (1991) *Theory and Nursing: a systematic approach.* St Louis, MO, Mosby.

Christie, F. (2007) Ongoing dialogue: functional linguistic and Bernsteinian sociological perspectives on education. In: F. Christie and J. R. Martin (eds) *Language, Knowledge and Pedagogy*. London, Continuum, pp.3–13.

Cowan, D. T., Norman, I. and Coopamah, V. P. (2005) Competence in nursing practice: a controversial concept; a focused review of the literature. *Nurse Education Today*, 25(5), 355–62.

Cowan, D. T., Wilson-Barnett, D. J., Norman, I. J., *et al.* (2007) Measuring nursing competence: development of a self-assessment tool for general nurses across Europe. *International Journal of Nursing Studies*, 45(6), 902–13.

Davies, B. (2001) Introduction. In: A. Morais, I. Neves and B. Davies (eds) *Towards a Sociology of Pedagogy: the contribution of Basil Bernstein to research*. New York, NY, Peter Lang, pp.1–14.

Dowling, P. (1999) *Basil Bernstein in Frame: 'Oh dear, is this a structuralist analysis?'* Available from: http://homepage.mac.com/paulcdowling/ioe/publications/kings1999/index.html (accessed 13 February 2011).

Dowling, P. (2001) Basil Bernstein: prophet, teacher, friend. In: S. Power (ed.) *A Tribute to Basil Bernstein, 1924–2000*. London, Institute of Education, University of London, pp.114–16.

Fisher, M. (2005) Exploring how nurse lecturers maintain clinical credibility. *Nurse Education in Practice*, 5(1), 21–9.

Gamble, J. (2004) Retrieving the general from the particular: the structure of craft knowledge. In: J. Muller, B. Davies and A. Morais (eds) *Reading Bernstein, Researching Bernstein*. London, RoutledgeFalmer, pp.189–203.

Gergen, K. A. (1985) Social constructivist enquiry: context and implications. In: K. A. Gergen and K. E. Davis (eds) *The Social Construction of the Person*. New York, NY, Springer-Verlag, pp.3–18.

Glen, S. (2004) Interprofessional education: the evidence base influencing policy and policy makers. *Nurse Education Today*, 24(3), 157–9.

Haigh, C. (2005) Where are the keynote debates in nurse education? *Nurse Education Today*, 25(5), 341–3.

Harré, R. and Secord, P. F. (1972) *The Explanation of Social Behaviour*. Oxford, Blackwell.

Hasan, R. (2004) The concept of semiotic perspectives: perspectives from Bernstein's sociology. In: J. Muller, B. Davies and A. Morais (eds) *Reading Bernstein, Researching Bernstein*. London, RoutledgeFalmer, pp.30–43.

Hill, Y., Lomas, L. and MacGregor, J. (2003) Managers, researchers teachers, and dabblers: enabling a research culture in nursing departments in higher education institutions. *Journal of Further and Higher Education*, 27(3), 317–31.

Johnson, M. (2004) What's wrong with nursing education research? *Nurse Education Today*, 24(8), 585–8.

Landers, M. G. (2000) The theory-practice gap in nursing: the role of the nurse teacher. *Journal of Advanced Nursing*, 32(6), 1550–56.

Maton, K. (2000) Languages of legitimation: the structuring significance for intellectual fields of strategic knowledge claims. *British Journal for the Sociology of Education*, 21(2), 147–67.

Maton, K. (2004) *The Field of Higher Education: a sociology of reproduction, transformation, change and the condition of emergence for cultural studies*. PhD thesis. University of Cambridge.

McNamara, M., Fealy, G. M., Casey, M., *et al.* (2011) Boundary matters: clinical leadership and the distinctive disciplinary contribution of nursing to multidisciplinary care. *Journal of Clinical Nursing*, 20(23–24), 3502–12.

McNamara, M. S. (2008) Of bedpans and ivory towers? Nurse academics' identities and the sacred and profane: a Bernsteinian analysis and discussion paper. *International Journal of Nursing Studies*, 45(3), 458–70.

McPherson, N. G. (2008) The role of sociology in nurse education: a call for consistency. *Nurse Education Today*, 28(6), 653–6.

Meirs, M. (2002) Nurse education in higher education: understanding cultural barriers to progress. *Nurse Education Today*, 22(3), 212–9.

Moore, R. (2006) Knowledge structures and intellect fields: Basil Bernstein and the sociology of knowledge. In: R. Moore, M. Arnot, J. Beck, *et al.* (eds) *Knowledge, Power and Educational Reform: applying the sociology of Basil Bernstein*. London, Routledge, pp.28–43.

Morais, A. and Neves, I. (2001) Pedagogic social contexts: studies for a sociology of learning In: A. Morais, I. Neves and B. Davies (eds) *Towards a Sociology of Pedagogy: the contribution of Basil Bernstein to research*. Oxford, Peter Lang, pp.185–221.

Muller, J. (2004) Introduction: the possibilities of Basil Bernstein. In: J. Muller, B. Davies and A. Morais (eds) *Reading Bernstein, Researching Bernstein*. London, RoutledgeFalmer, pp.1–12.

Nolan, M., Ingleton, C. and Hayter, M. (2008) The Research Excellence Framework (REF): a major impediment to free and informed debate? *International Journal of Nursing Studies*, 45(4), 487–8.

Norman, I. J., Watson, R., Murrells, T., *et al.* (2002) The validity and reliability of methods to assess the competence to practice of pre-registration nursing and midwifery students. *International Journal of Nursing Studies*, 39(2), 133–45.

O'Connor, S. J. (2007) Developing professional habitus: a Bernsteinian analysis of the modern nurse apprenticeship. *Nurse Education Today*, 27(7), 748–54.

Parse, R. R. (1998) *The Human Becoming School of Thought: a perspective for nurses and other health professionals*. Thousand Oaks, CA, Sage.

Parse, R. R. (2008) Nursing knowledge development: who's to say how? *Nursing Science Quarterly*, 21(2), 101.

Porter, S. (1995) Sociology and the nursing curriculum: a defence. *Journal of Advanced Nursing*, 21(6), 1130–35.

Rafferty, A. M., Allcock, N. and Lathlean, J. (1996) The theory/practice gap: taking issue with the issue. *Journal of Advanced Nursing*, 23(4), 685–91.

Ramsden, P. (1992) *Learning to Teach in Higher Education*. London, Routledge.

Reay, D. (2004) Cultural capitalists and academic habitus: classed and gendered labour in UK higher education. *Women's Studies International Forum*, 27(1), 31–9.

Rolfe, G. and Freshwater, D. (2005) To save the honour of thinking: a slightly petulant response to Griffiths. *International Journal of Nursing Studies*, 42(3), 363–9.

Sabin, M. (2001) *Competence in Practice-based Calculation: issues for nurse education; a critical review of the literature*. London, Learning, Teaching and Support Network for Health Science and Practice.

Sandelowski, M. (1986) The problem of rigor in qualitative research. *American Nursing Society Advances in Nursing Science*, 8(3), 27–37.

Sharp, K. (1994) Sociology and the nursing curriculum: a note of caution. *Journal of Advanced Nursing*, 20(2), 391–5.

Sharp, K. (1995) Sociology in nurse education: help or hindrance? *Nursing Times*, 91(20), 34–5.

Shotter, J. (1993) *Cultural Politics of Everyday Life: social constructivism, rhetoric and knowing of the third kind*. Buckingham, Open University Press.

Thomas, E. and Davies, B. (2006) Nurse teachers' knowledge in curriculum planning and implementation. *Nurse Education Today*, 26(7), 572–7.

Walford, G. (1995) Classification and framing in English public boarding schools. In: P. Atkinson, B. Davies, S. Delamont, *et al.* (eds) *Discourse and Reproduction: essays in honor of Basil Bernstein*. Creskill, NJ, Hampton, pp.147–58.

Walsh, C. L., Gordon, M. F., Marshall, M., *et al.* (2005) Interprofessional capability: a developing framework for interprofessional education. *Nurse Education in Practice*, 5(4), 230–37.

5

From classroom to clinic

An activity theory perspective

Clare Morris

JUST OVER A DECADE AGO, THE UK GENERAL MEDICAL COUNCIL produced a guidance document called *The Doctor as Teacher* (GMC, 1999), beginning what could be viewed as the 'professionalisation' of medical education (Swanwick, 2009; Eitel *et al.*, 2000). *The Doctor as Teacher* made clear the professional obligation of all doctors to contribute to the education of others on the team, noted that teaching skills can be learnt and stipulated that doctors with teaching responsibilities should take steps to ensure the development of their teaching skills. Since then, increasing attention has been paid to the development of doctors as teachers; 'faculty development' is becoming a shared concern of medical schools and network organisations in the National Health Service (NHS) that have been established specifically to manage and deliver postgraduate medical training (the NHS Deaneries) (Swanwick, 2009). Masters-level courses in medical education have proliferated (Pugsley *et al.*, 2008) and professional regulators have become increasingly concerned with the need to define standards for medical trainers and training (GMC, 2010; PMETB, 2006). Within academic medical institutions, this type of development activity has been relatively common, linked to an expectation that academic staff should be versed in curriculum design and in teaching, learning and assessment strategies. The significance of the General Medical Council guidance is that this expectation has extended from the academy into clinical workplaces and into the teaching activity of clinicians.

It was within this changing context that one large London-based medical school extended its work activity to specifically encompass faculty development for academics and clinicians engaged in supporting the learning of their undergraduates. As the new postholder, I was anxious to identify the ways in which I could work with colleagues to help them develop their education and training practices. Although from a clinical background, I was relatively new to medical education and was keen to identify what might be considered 'best practice' within the classrooms of the medical school and in the wards, clinics and theatres where medical students undertook their clinical attachments (this research commenced in 2004, before the major reform of UK postgraduate medical education).

The existing medical education literatures seemed mainly to focus on 'how to teach' or on the responsibilities of medical educators of different grades (GMC, 1999, 1997, 1993). There appeared to be little consideration of the cultures of medical education or the theoretical underpinnings of medical education practice (Morris, 2009). It was from this starting point. therefore, that I set out to 'make sense' of pedagogic practices across the medical school I worked in. My goal was to move beyond ideas of *how* to teach, to explore *why* doctors may choose to teach in particular ways.

Making sense of medical education: the role of activity theory

An early research decision was to draw upon Engeström's third-generation activity theory (Engeström, 2001) in order to theorise the medical school. Daniels (2009), a researcher within the traditions of activity theory, notes that: 'theory is not understood as an immutable given, rather it is understood as a repository of tools for engaging with contemporary problems' (p.260). I had been introduced to activity theory during my doctoral studies and felt it offered the rich 'repository of tools' needed when seeking to research medical education. These tools take the form of five guiding principles that invite the researcher to analyse 'activity' within and across organisations in particular ways. In my case, they suggested a way of analysing the activity of medical education across higher education and NHS organisational settings.

Later in this chapter, some of this analysis is shared as a way of illustrating the potential value of activity theory in medical education research. However, in order to understand the guiding principles of this theory and how they may be put to use, it is necessary to look first at the ways in which activity theory challenges dominantly held views about learning and invites educational researchers to engage in a type of rethinking, described by Arnseth (2008) as:

> stepping away from taking social structures or individual cognition as the primary constituents of the orderliness of educational phenomena. … social practices are and should be the primary objects of inquiry. (p.289)

In other words, to move beyond researching individuals, their practices or perspectives, to researching shared practices in context. In activity theory, this means looking not only at enacted practices (the activity) but also at the object of this activity. When Engeström uses the term 'activity', he is referencing particular social practices that, in simple terms, include not only what someone is 'doing', but the human will and intention behind the 'doing' (Arnseth, 2008). While activity theory can be seen to share many similarities with other socio-cultural views on learning (particularly situated learning theory), there are notable differences, not least in terms of the intended goal of learning. Sfard (1998) draws our attention to the distinctions between two guiding metaphors for learning. In learning-as-acquisition, the goal of any learning activity is framed in terms of the acquisition of knowledge and skills. Learning-as-participation (deriving from socio-cultural theories of learning) sees the goal of any learning activity being full participation in the practices of a community. If we were to offer a third metaphor, derived from activity theory, it might be learning-as-expansion (Morris, 2011). In activity theory, therefore, the goal is expansive transformation of systems (which includes the situated practices of actors in that system, but also the system itself). These types of expansive transformations are understood in terms of the collective, deliberative change efforts that can come about as the result of tensions arising within the system itself. An example might be the tension many clinical teachers face, between allowing students and trainees to 'practise' on patients and meeting a duty of care to the patients to ensure their safety and optimal care. Therefore, a question arises as to the ways in which clinical teachers develop their practice (as educators) to reconcile these tensions. Historically, closely supervised practice may be one response. In more recent times, simulated practice may be seen as another response to this tension.

In activity theory, social practices are seen as object-oriented activity – that is, activity with an attached purpose. This perspective would therefore lead us not only to explore what clinical teachers 'do' when they engage students in the ward round, for example, but the intended purposes of their activity. Teaching here becomes more than an act (be it asking questions, examining patients and so forth); it becomes an activity aimed at preparing medical students for their future roles as doctors. This preparation may move beyond a focus on the acquisition of certain types of knowledge or skill sets, to the shaping of ways of thinking, being and acting as doctors. Making sense of medical education therefore extends beyond observable teaching behaviours or strategies, towards the explicit and implicit purposes shaping these practices.

Activity theory builds upon the work of Vygotsky (1978), who originally provided the triangular model of mediated human action (subject – mediating tools – object) on which it is based. In this model, action consists of a *subject* (the actor), an *object* (goal-oriented activity) and *meditational tools*, which can be either material or conceptual. Figure 5.1 provides a representation of ward round teaching, using this model. The action of teaching during a ward round can be represented by the subject (the medical teacher) seeking to prepare future doctors for their roles (the object) through case-based discussions, examination of patients and analysis of patient charts and data (the mediating tools). The mediated nature of this activity is an important facet of activity theory. For example, when clinical teachers 'teach' on the ward round, they will draw upon a range of mediating tools or artefacts which are embedded in the activity. These may be symbolic or conceptual tools (e.g. specialist terminology and/or mnemonics) as well as material tools. For example, a stethoscope may mediate the act of learning to listen for breath sounds or heartbeats, an electrocardiogram trace may mediate the act of learning how to recognise a myocardial infarction, a patient may mediate the act of learning to take a history. In addition to their mediating function as a teaching tool, such artefacts often have historical cultural significance in the activity system; this is discussed in more detail later in this chapter.

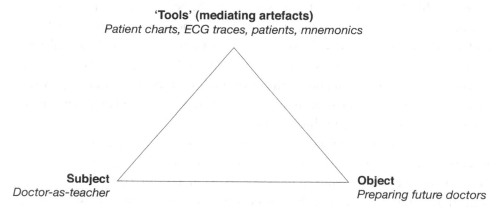

FIGURE 5.1 Ward round teaching as mediated activity

Engeström (1999) takes Vygotsky's model (so-called first-generation activity theory) one step further, moving beyond an individual to a collective focus on the activity system. Human activity is understood as being embedded within particular activity systems, each with their own rules, communities and divisions of labour. Figure 5.2 provides a representation of the ward round as an activity system. Here, the original triangular model is extended. The *community* of an activity system encompasses those who share the object of the activity, for example, patient care or medical training. *Divisions of labour* are understood in terms of the ways in which particular tasks, activities and benefits are distributed among community members engaged in the shared activity. *Rules* are both explicit and implicit, determining and shaping the ways in which activity is realised. If second-generation activity theory is used to analyse ward round teaching, such teaching could be understood as a mediated activity that takes place in a complex system, with identifiable traditions (the ward round being one of these), practices (examination of patients, case presentations), rules ('business before teaching'), roles (nurses 'care', doctors 'cure') and cultures (surgical rounds being 'different' from medical rounds, for example).

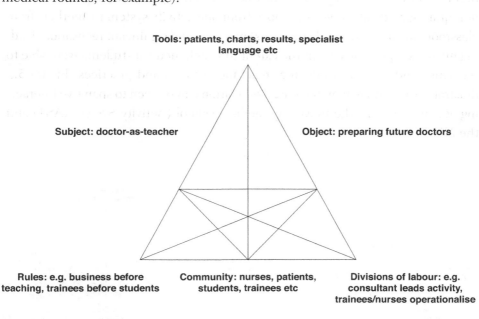

FIGURE 5.2 The ward round as an activity system (note: 'trainee' is used here and elsewhere in the chapter to refer to a doctor who has completed undergraduate medical training and first professional registration but who is still undertaking the training for full specialist registration)

Third-generation activity theory

However, medical students do not just learn within the clinical environment; their experiences of being taught span a wide range of contexts, including those within the medical school. In a study seeking to make sense of medical education, an analytic framework that goes beyond a single system, however complex, is merited. This is where Engeström's 'third-generation activity theory' offers a way forward, extending the unit of analysis from one to at least two interacting activity systems (Engeström, 2001).

A pivotal point in my research study was recognising that the institution of the 'medical school' was best understood as two interacting activity systems: the university-based medical school and the NHS-based clinical attachments. While participants in each system may share medical education as an object of their activity, the ways in which they mediate this activity and the contexts and communities in which it happens are distinct. Rethinking the learning implications of requiring medical students to move from one activity system to another (from classroom to clinic, in simplistic terms) was a second significant realisation, leading me to ask questions about the extent to which medical students were able to recognise and respond to distinct teaching cultures and practices. Figure 5.3 illustrates the ways in which medical education can be seen to span two interacting activity systems: the university medical school (Activity System (AS1) and the NHS (AS2)).

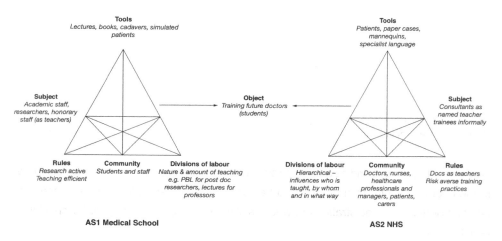

FIGURE 5.3 The medical school as two interacting activity systems

Putting the guiding principles of activity theory to use
• • • • • • • • • •

The five guiding principles of activity theory (the theoretical tools) (Engeström, 1999) were used as a framework to analyse the medical school as an AS. Each of these five principles is briefly explained here, before being illustrated with examples taken from my analysis of the medical school (see Morris, 2009). The first principle concerns the identification of the unit of analysis for research, which has to be at least two *interacting activity systems* (in this case, the medical school (AS1) and the NHS (AS2)). The second principle is the *multi-voicedness* of activity systems, which comprise '*a community of multiple points of view, traditions and interest*' (Engeström 1999). Third is the importance of *historicity* when analysing activity systems. Engeström (1999) notes that activity systems develop and transform over long periods; they can only be understood by undertaking a historical analysis of the theoretical ideas and tools that have shaped their activity. The fourth principle is recognising historically accumulating *contradictions* and tensions as creative sources for change and development of systems (and therefore the activity of those systems). The final principle is the possibility of *expansive transformations* of activity systems, with deliberative collective change efforts having the potential to radically change the object of the activity system and its purpose. In activity theory, learning is seen as a distributed phenomenon, arising from interactions between individuals, their colleagues and the conceptual and physical tools that are used; learning goes beyond the individual to the activity system itself. These five guiding principles offered a way into my analysis of the medical school, allowing me to theorise the institution-in-focus for my doctoral studies and develop research questions for later fieldwork (*see* Chapter 1).

The aim of my analysis was to make sense of the pedagogic practices being adopted by academics and clinical teachers and the ways in which medical students experienced these practices. This started with a process of analysing each system, identifying shared and distinct practices within and across them. In this way, I aimed to use the principles as theoretical tools in order to analyse the interactions between 'classroom and clinic'. In doing this, I drew upon a range of sources and experiences, including my own biographical resources. I had a developing understanding of organisational practices and purposes. I was engaged in peer observation of teaching practices as part of my work activity; this yielded powerful insights into medical teaching practices both in the medical school and in medical workplaces. I spent time reading and thinking through organisational documents, which guided or reported on curriculum, teaching and learning principles and practices; this included student and tutor handbooks supporting clinical attachments. Importantly, my ongoing faculty development work offered rich opportunities to talk about teaching, learning and assessment practices with staff from each activity system, as well as those who worked in both. I was particularly concerned with the ways in which teaching practices were problematical and the types of frustrations expressed (as these may be the types of 'tensions' that lead to innovation in working practices). This analysis was an iterative and ongoing process, further shaped by later fieldwork, where I observed and talked to medical students about their learning experiences. Reporting the complete analysis of the medical school is beyond the scope of this chapter; however, parts of the analysis are presented here to illustrate the analytical value of activity theory.

Principle one: a collective unit of analysis

A key concern for any educational researcher is the need to identify the most appropriate unit for analysis, the *scholarly creations* that enable theoretical perspectives to be put to use (Säljö, 2009, 2007). In activity theory, the first guiding principle predetermines the unit of analysis as interacting 'artefact-mediated and object-orientated' activity systems (Engeström, 2004). This leads to explicit consideration of shared activity across systems, including the conceptualisation of 'boundary objects' and 'boundary crossing'. In conceptualising the medical school as two interacting activity systems with a shared object of activity, it was possible to construct a richer, more nuanced account of the pedagogic practices employed within and across systems. For example, while the curriculum of the medical school had been influenced by the guidance provided by the General Medical Council (1993) in *Tomorrow's Doctors*, it had retained a traditional technocratic structure, with an observable preclinical–clinical divide. Learning in the early years was largely based within the university medical school (AS1), mediated by lectures, tutorials and anatomy sessions. Learning in the later years was increasingly based within the NHS (AS2), mediated by bedside teaching, ward rounds and patients. However, closer analysis identified boundary crossing mediating artefacts, e.g. communication skills sessions with 'simulated patients' (actors) within the university medical school (AS1) or simulated patient-care experiences within skills centres in the NHS (AS2).

It is important to recognise that each individual activity system within the unit of analysis has competing objects. In the university medical school (AS1), academic staff are expected not only to prepare future doctors but also to engage in types of research activity that will attract external funding and increase reputational resource. In the NHS (AS2), doctors are expected not only to prepare future doctors but also to meet service demands and deliver high-quality patient care. Potential tensions between the dual objects of each system are likely to arise. For example, in the NHS (AS2), the desire to offer medical students authentic, hands-on patient care experiences is balanced with a focus on patient safety and service efficiency. In my analysis of the medical school, explicit noting of these structural tensions was important, informing my interpretation of both historical and newly emerging pedagogic practices.

Principle two: multi-voicedness

Engeström (2004) notes that activity systems

> are always a community of multiple points of view, traditions and interests ... The multi-voicedness is multiplied in networks of interacting activity systems. It is a source of trouble and innovations, demanding actions of translation and negotiation. (p.149)

In analysing the medical school, attention was paid to the different 'voices' expressed through the design of curriculum and the choice of teaching practices adopted across each system. Some voices were more dominant than others. For example, in the university medical school (AS1), the voices of senior clinical academic staff (professoriate, department leads) were heard more loudly than those of postdoctoral researchers or students themselves when decisions were made about how to organise teaching, learning and assessment practices. The voice of the General Medical Council was evident in changes to curriculum practices and the voices of clinicians from the NHS (AS2) were also influential to some degree; in order to offer a medical qualification, the school has to ensure a suitable range of clinical placement experiences for students. My analysis of the institution therefore had to be actively sensitive to possible competing 'views, traditions and interests' and look for signs of how these were played out in adopted pedagogic practices, divisions of (teaching) labour and the 'rules' of the system, embedded in curriculum models, student handbooks and so forth.

The way in which problem-based learning (PBL) was adopted into the curriculum of the medical school provided an example of how competing 'views, traditions and interests' played out in adopting pedagogic practices. In 1993, the General Medical Council published *Tomorrow's Doctors*, a guidance document with an intended purpose of curriculum regeneration in undergraduate medical education. The extent to which medical schools responded to the guidance within the document was monitored through quality assurance visits, which in turn determined whether the school continued to award primary medical qualifications. Therefore medical schools were arguably required to respond favourably to this request. Within this first version of *Tomorrow's Doctors* was a strong steer to reduce the traditional technocratic structure of the undergraduate curriculum. Early patient contact was encouraged, along with an integrated, systems-based curriculum and the adoption of problem-based learning. Many of the new medical schools being created in the United Kingdom at the time adopted this guidance wholesale. However, for established medical schools, with long histories of organising their curriculum in a different way, i.e. terms of preclinical university-based and then clinical hospital-based stages, with strongly teacher-led pedagogic practices (such as expert lectures), this guidance was a potential source of both 'trouble' and 'innovation'.

Therefore, the established medical school that was the location of this research study found itself in a 'contradictory positioning', in activity theory terms. It had long-established traditions that it wished to retain, yet it had to make changes to meet the requirements of the General Medical Council (and therefore the continuity of the activity system). An analysis of its response to the adoption of PBL is revealing, when understood in these terms. The school undertook a major curriculum reform, creating an explicit (yet thin) PBL 'strand' in the curriculum, most visible in the first 2 years of the course. However, much of the strongly technocratic organisational division of teaching remained even after the introduction of PBL. Closer analysis of the implementation of this curriculum strand was revealing, in terms of division of labour. Few of the established university medical school (AS1) academic staff were involved in PBL; they continued to use historical teaching practices such as lectures. PBL sessions, which were apparently unpopular with both academic staff and students, were frequently delegated to postdoctoral researchers (often framed in terms of an opportunity for them to gain entry into future academic posts) and clinical staff from the NHS (AS2), who were rewarded with honorary posts within the university medical school (AS1).

Thus, in tracing the school's response to the General Medical Council guidance using activity theory, my attention was drawn to the uneven distribution of teaching practices (divisions of labour) and the changing constitution of the teaching faculty (community). It became much clearer, to me at least, that different teaching practices within and across the system, held different statuses. This closer, activity theory based analysis led me to think differently about the faculty I could be working with and the types of teaching activity each might be engaged in. It also led me to think about how the perceived status of different types of teaching and learning experiences might influence student engagement with these.

Principle three: historicity

Engeström (2004) remarks: 'the activity system itself carries multiple layers of history, engraved in its artifacts, rules and conventions' (p.149). In an activity theory based analysis, it is important to seek to understand how particular forms of activity arise and are realised. The medical school's response to the adoption of PBL (with resulting divisions of labour and changes in the community) can only be understood with some appreciation of what has happened in the past. This third principle of historicity means recognising that activity systems take shape over long periods, and that participants within systems will bring their own history to bear on their activities. In my analysis of the medical school, there were signs that new forms of teaching activity were regarded less favourably (by academic staff at least) than those historically established. This led to uneven distribution of teaching labour and new subjects being brought into the system. Within the university medical school (AS1), for example, the preparation of future doctors includes the use of longstanding, historically recognised teaching activities, including professorial lectures and dissection and prosection of cadavers. In the NHS (AS2), the traditions of clinical medicine (which date back to the time of the French Revolution) are seen in the ward round and bedside teaching sessions. Teaching activities of more recent provenance are also present in both systems. The teaching of communication skills involving 'simulated patients' as mediating artefacts in the university medical school (AS1), or the teaching of procedural skills using manikins in dedicated clinical skills centres (often led by nursing staff) within the NHS (AS2) are cases in point.

A closer analysis of the history of communication skills teaching, which again was foregrounded by the GMC (1993) guidance, illustrates how teaching activities develop over time (i.e. historically) in response to contradictions and tensions in the activity systems. Historically, the development of clinical communication skills could be seen as part of the implicit curriculum of the NHS (AS2). The students built their communication skills iteratively, in context, through working within medical teams and with patients. A process of curriculum reform has now made communication skills teaching an explicit strand of the curriculum, taught almost entirely by psychologists working with simulated patients (trained actors). This new form of teaching activity within the medical school meets the General Medical Council requirements and perhaps becomes another boundary object for medical students, who are expected to translate their learning of communication skills (taught by non-clinicians with proxy patients) into engagements with clinicians and patients who may, in reality, communicate quite differently. Understanding the arrival of new mediating artefacts and practices leads us to the fourth principle of activity theory, the central role of contradictions as sources of change and development.

Principle four: the central role of contradictions

Engeström (2004) describes activity systems as 'virtual disturbance-and-innovation-producing machines' (p.150), explicitly arguing for the creative potential of contradictions within and across activity systems. In using the term 'contradictions', he is clear in differentiating them from problems, describing the former as historically accumulating structural tensions, which by necessity will lead to changes in activity and expansions of activity systems. Examples of my analysis of AS1 illustrate ways in which the academic community responded to the contradictory positioning arising from the changing General Medical Council guidance on the purposes, structure and pedagogic practices to be realised within the system. New forms of activity are evident, each carrying different entailments in terms of who leads the activity and the divisions of labour across the system.

In analysing the NHS (AS2), it was possible to identify contradictions and creative responses to them in the form of new mediating tools and teaching activities. At the time of my study, clinical skills centres were being created and, in some teaching hospitals, opportunities to engage in high-fidelity simulation were appearing. In my analysis, newly emerging pedagogic practices were understood as a response to the contradictory positioning that clinical teachers found themselves in as a result of NHS reform. Historically, medical student and trainee learning in the workplace has been integral to participation in working activity. Students were given hands-on learning experiences of increasing complexity during clinical placements, they shadowed qualified doctors during rotations and they were then given junior doctor roles immediately after qualification. These types of learning experiences took place in established work teams (often described as 'clinical firms') who were able to 'safety-net' the work of less experienced firm members.

Changes in NHS (AS2) organisation led to the fragmentation of clinical firms into much larger, looser teams based on or around clinical specialities. Developments in technology have meant that patients stay in hospital for shorter periods, and there has been an increased focus on performance efficiency. There has also been a shift in culture toward a greater emphasis on patient rights and safety. In these changing contexts, learning-through-work in the NHS (AS2) has become a less viable strategy. Thus simulation training can be seen as a creative, innovative response to the contradictory positioning that clinical staff occupy. In activity theory terms, simulation becomes a boundary object, supporting transitions 'from classroom to clinic'.

Principle five: the possibility of expansive transformation of systems

Engeström (1999) distinguishes between the long cycles of transformation that occur over time and those arising from deliberative change efforts that occur when individuals begin to question established practices and move away from them. Deliberative change efforts involve the adoption of interventionist research practices that actively bring together individuals from across an activity system to undertake a purposeful analysis of that system. This analysis identifies the structurally accumulating tensions that leave them in the types of contradictory positions illustrated earlier. This leads to a collective envisioning of different ways of operating that are taken back into the system and subsequently reviewed. This approach takes participants through an expansive learning cycle. My activity theory led analysis of the medical school as two interactive activity systems in essence, followed through this analytical cycle. Using the principle of expansive transformations analytically in my own work was helpful in identifying significant shifts in teaching, learning and assessment practices within and across both activity systems. The identification of changed or developing practices led me to consider the creative tensions behind them. It also led me to think about the extent to which academic and clinical teachers felt engaged with new approaches and comfortable in their adoption. This was immediately significant to my work as a faculty developer within and across activity systems.

Medical education as boundary-crossing activity

Figure 5.3 provides a diagrammatic representation of the medical school as two interacting systems, based on the analysis undertaken (partially represented in this chapter). In developing my analysis, I started to conceptualise medical students as boundary crossers who engaged with the object of both systems, to different extents at different stages of their education and training. For example, medical students spend the early years of their study based within the university medical school (AS1). As students progress within the course, they spend more time within the NHS (AS2). Students have to learn to make sense of the pedagogic practices adopted in both activity systems, from the historically recognised to the newly emerging. Increasingly, they experience teaching away from patients (real and simulated), as pedagogic practices more familiar in the university medical school (AS1) (such as lectures and seminars) seep into the NHS clinical workplaces (AS2). I was able to pick up the extent to which they were able to do this in later fieldwork.

For some students (particularly those in the early years of their course), the ability to recognise the types of learning embedded in the everyday activity of their clinical attachments was problematic and clinical teachers were not always ready to make them explicit. This is another example of clinical teachers finding themselves in a contradictory positioning. Do they try and make explicit the learning inherent in working, or respond by providing the types of learning experiences that students recognise from their time spent in the university medical school (AS1)? This analysis suggests possible ways forward for faculty development activity. Rather than teaching doctors to be 'better teachers', there is a case to be made for helping doctors make the learning embedded in practice more explicit.

My activity theory based analysis led me to question much more actively the role and purposes of faculty development work within and across the medical school. I began to conceptualise my work in much more nuanced ways, recognising that pedagogic practices were distinct, with long histories of practice behind them. Therefore, in developing my own activity I had to be mindful of a need to support and develop both medical academics (in the university medical school – AS1) and doctors-as-teachers (in the NHS – AS2) in ways that were culturally and contextually sensitive. The identification of tensions and contradictions within and across systems invited consideration of the potential to innovate in teaching, learning and assessment practices. It also suggested the need to be aware of and responsive to the ways in which the teachers in the two activity systems were able to reconcile the sometimes competing objects of activity of their respective activity systems. The identification of a broad range of pedagogic practices also raised questions about the ways in which medical students were able to make sense of and engage with the learning opportunities that were both explicitly and implicitly available in each system.

Through theorising the medical school in these ways, it was possible for me to identify and deconstruct the multiple voices and the contradictions that made up its whole. My initial desire to make sense of the wide-ranging pedagogic practices adopted within and across the medical school was undoubtedly aided by looking through an activity theory 'lens'. Teaching practices were understood in terms of their historicity and the multiple (and often competing) interests of community members. Newly emerging practices were understood as innovation in times of disturbance and turbulence. This, in turn, led me to identify the logical next step for my study, which was to identify the NHS (AS2) as the primary unit of analysis for more in-depth study of medical student learning (*see* Chapter 1).

Working across boundaries

In seeking to make sense of medical education in my own institution, the challenges faced by medical students as boundary crossers became apparent. Given the opportunities I had to bring their 'teachers' together, this led me to question established faculty development practices and think differently about how I might work in the future. The research undertaken led me to rethink faculty development in a number of ways.

The first was to consider the extent to which it was possible to identify a single coherent pedagogy to underpin the work of doctors as teachers. Given the organisational complexity, the different epistemological positions of community members and the wide range of teaching, learning and assessment practices observed, this seemed unlikely. It is possible to argue the need for doctors-as-teachers to examine the thinking that underpins their practices, and part of this means offering a range of theoretical tools that may allow them to do this. The second was to consider how best to balance the development needs of different members of each activity system and how to bring value to faculty development sessions which involved members from each. For example, those in the university medical school (AS1) desired opportunities to appreciate the thinking behind the adoption of problem-based learning and to hone skills in facilitation, while those in the NHS (AS2) were keen to explore how to make best use of new mediating tools offered in clinical skills centres. However, in faculty development sessions where teachers from each system came together, opportunities could be harnessed to open up a critical dialogue between those who shared the 'development of future doctors' as an object of activity. By exploring their historically established cultural practices, it might be possible to find ways to innovate practices in the rapidly changing worlds in which each was operating. This approach follows similar principles to Engeström's change laboratory work, where problems are brought into close focus and practitioners work collectively to think through and try out new ways of working (Engeström, 2007).

The third rethinking recognised the rich resources that medical students as boundary crossers may bring to faculty development activity. In the research study undertaken, it was clear that medical students recognised the ways in which some teachers, more than others, invited them into their workplaces, creating opportunities to learn through engagement in the day-to-day activity of the workplace. These teachers were able to make explicit the learning embedded in daily work activity and did not seek refuge in teaching strategies more relevant to the academy. Rethinking faculty development may mean inviting a much more active engagement of medical students to help mediate the learning of their teachers.

Moving beyond the limitations of activity theory

The research study used as an exemplar in this chapter was undertaken in 2004. Although Engeström had been engaged in researching medical practices in Finland (Engeström, 1993) it was not possible, at the time, to identify studies where activity theory had been used to research medical education, either within the United Kingdom or elsewhere. Bleakley (2006) subsequently encouraged medical education researchers to consider using activity theory to understand distributed and complex practices within medical teams. However, at the time of my study, there was little debate in the literatures about the ways in which educational researchers might deploy the tools of activity theory in their own research to achieve such outcomes. Engeström's own work adopts interventionist methodologies, with particular intents to expand practices. His change laboratory methodology seeks to identify contradictions and then foster the types of collective envisioning that lead to change (and expansive learning). This approach, even if resources had been available, was not aligned to the object of my own research activity, which was to make sense of the pedagogic practices of clinical teachers and the types of educational conceptual tools they might usefully draw upon. It was, however, possible to put the guiding principles of activity theory to use in a purposeful analysis of the medical school. The conceptualisation of the medical school as two interacting activity systems, for example, invited a much more nuanced and purposeful analysis of observed pedagogic practices and how they acted on the object of activity, the training of future doctors. The identification of tensions and contradictions offered a way to make sense of newly emerging forms of pedagogic practice and mediating tools during the period of my study.

However, as a researcher new to activity theory, I found it difficult to operationalise these principles in subsequent fieldwork investigating medical student learning in the workplace. My analysis of the medical school influenced the framing of my research questions for this fieldwork, but it did not offer me a way into designing or defining methodology and methods. More recently, Daniels *et al.* (2010) have noted the ways in which researchers seeking to work within the traditions of activity theory see it as: 'a developing resource encompassing core principles, yet flexibly responsive to fields of study' (p.1). Looking back at my research work, it is possible to identify how activity theory principles were used flexibly to theorise my institution and to make sense of pedagogic practices. This led me to ask questions of the ways in which medical students made sense of teaching, learning and assessment practices within and across the system and the extent to which they were invited to engage with those experiences in meaningful ways. Arnseth (2008), in his excellent critique of the similarities and differences between activity theory and situated learning theory suggests that used together, these two approaches provide powerful internal and external perspectives on human practices. In my own work, activity theory and socio-cultural theories allowed a critique of medical education that led me to think differently about faculty development and develop my practice accordingly. Activity theory offers new ways of thinking about medical learning and practice. By drawing upon the tools offered, I was able to 'theorise' the medical school I worked within and critically analyse the teaching and learning practices observed. This provided a way forward in terms of rethinking faculty development practices. Ultimately, this research work has had a significant impact on the ways in which I work with medical, dental and healthcare educators in undergraduate and postgraduate settings and the theoretical tools and resources I bring to bear on my activity as a faculty developer and academic.

References

Arnseth, H. (2008) Activity theory and situated learning theory: contrasting views of educational practice. *Pedagogy, Culture and Society*, 16(3), 289–302.

Bleakley, A. (2006) Broadening conceptions of learning in medical education: the message from team-working. *Medical Education*, 40(2), 150–7.

Daniels, H. (2009) Introduction to section 5: deploying theory. In: H. Daniels, H. Lauder and J. Porter (eds) *Knowledge, Values and Educational Policy: a critical perspective*. Oxford, Routledge, pp.261–2.

Daniels, H., Edwards, A., Engeström, Y., *et al.* (eds) (2010) *Activity Theory in Practice: promoting learning across boundaries and agencies*. London, Routledge.

Eitel, F., Kanz, K. and Tesche, A. (2000) Training and certification of teachers and trainers: the professionalization of medical education. *Medical Teacher*, 22(5), 517–26.

Engeström, Y. (1993) Developmental studies on work as a test bench of AT. In: Chaiklin, S and Lave, J. *Understanding Practice: perspectives on activity and context*. Cambridge, Cambridge University Press, pp.64–103.

Engeström, Y. (1999) Innovative learning in work teams: analysing cycles of knowledge creation in practice. In: Y. Engeström, R. Miettinen and R. Punamaki (eds) *Perspectives on Activity Theory*. Cambridge, Cambridge University Press, pp.377–406.

Engeström, Y. (2001) Expansive learning at work: toward an activity theoretical reconceptualization. *Journal of Education and Work*, 14(1), 133–56.

Engeström, Y. (2004) The new generation of expertise: seven theses. In: H. Rainbird, A. Fuller and A. Munro (eds) *Workplace Learning in Context*. Oxford, Routledge, pp.145–65.

Engeström, Y. (2007) Putting Vygotsky to work: the change laboratory as an application of double simulation. In: H. Daniels, M. Cole and J. V. Wertsch (eds) *The Cambridge Companion to Vygotsky*. Cambridge, Cambridge University Press, pp.363–82.

General Medical Council (GMC) (1993) *Tomorrow's Doctors*. 1st edn. Available from: www.gmc-uk.org/Tomorrows_Doctors_1993.pdf_25397206.pdf (accessed 26 February 2011).

General Medical Council (GMC) (1997) *The New Doctor*. London, GMC.

General Medical Council (GMC) (1999) *The Doctor as Teacher: archived policy document*. Available from: www.gmc-uk.org/education/postgraduate/doctor_as_teacher.asp (accessed 20 April 2011).

General Medical Council (GMC) (2010) *Generic Standards for Specialty Including GP Training*. London, GMC.

Morris, C. (2009) Developing pedagogy for doctors-as-teachers: the role of activity theory. In: H. Daniels, H. Lauder and J. Porter (eds) *Knowledge, Values and Educational Policy: a critical perspective*. Oxford, Routledge, pp.273–81.

Morris, C. (2011) *From Time-served Apprenticeship to Time-measured Training: new challenges for postgraduate medical education*. Thesis submitted in partial fulfilment of the EdD, Institute of Education, University of London. October 2011.

Postgraduate Medical Education and Training Board (PMETB) (2006) *Generic Standards for Training*. London: PMETB.

Pugsley, L., Brigley, S., Allery, L., *et al.* (2008) Making a difference: researching masters and doctoral research programmes in medical education. *Medical Education*, 42(2), 157–63.

Säljö, R. (2007) *Studying Learning and Knowing in Social Practices: units of analysis and tensions in theorising*. Lecture given on the occasion of the opening of the Oxford Centre for Socio-cultural Activity Theory Research. Oxford, UK.

Säljö, R. (2009) Learning, theories of learning, and units of analysis in research. *Educational Psychologist*, 44(3), 202–8.

Sfard, A. (1998) On two metaphors for learning and the dangers of choosing just one. *Educational Researcher*, 27(1), 4–13.

Swanwick, T. (2009) Editorial: teaching the teachers: no longer an optional extra. *British Journal of Hospital Medicine*, 70(3), 176–7.

Vygotsky, L. S. (1978) *Mind in Society: development of higher psychological processes*, ed. and trans. M. Cole, Cambridge, MA, Harvard University Press.

6

'The hidden curriculum'

Learning the tacit and embodied nature of nursing practice

Mary Gobbi

THIS CHAPTER ARGUES THAT SOMETIMES WHEN RESEARCHING INTO aspects of clinical education and the 'nitty-gritty' of nursing practice, no single methodological or theoretical stance will suffice. Perhaps ironically, if there were only one methodological stance, it would be easier to generate a single universal theory to explain the multifaceted nuances of professional education. The chapter will explore the dilemmas raised by investigating how registered nurses learn and develop in daily clinical practice, with specific reference to their use of intuition, thinking and reflection-in-action. These study concepts are slippery, contested and multifaceted, with their universality and existence questioned. To investigate them, I need to confront the legacy of dualism (which means, in this case, the separation of mind from body in both thought and language), venture into the murky world of tacit embodied practice, address the links among thinking, doing, seeing and speaking, and to analyse these concepts with respect to existing theories concerning learning in professional practice. Selecting a method of investigation is not without its challenges when deciding how to investigate phenomena related to intuition and reflection-in-action. Ironically, Plato (1966) outlined these paradoxes in what is known as Meno's dilemma:

> But how will you look for something when you don't know what it is? How on earth are you going to set up something you don't know as the object of your search? To put it another way, even if you come up right against it, how will

you know that what you have found is the thing you didn't know? (Meno to Socrates, p.128)

Later, in response, Socrates outlined Meno's trick question:

He would not seek what he knows, for since he knows it there is not need of the inquiry, nor what he does not know, for in that case he does not even know what he is to look for. (p.129)

To manage these paradoxes, the study presented in the second part of this chapter needed to be hermeneutical, exploratory and pragmatic without compromising rigour in order to address Meno's questions, namely:

- How would I look for intuition, reflection and/or thinking-in-action if I don't know what it is (they are)?
- How will I set up something I don't know as the object of my search?
- How will I recognise intuition, reflection and/or thinking-in-action should I come right up against them (it)?

This chapter relates how conceptual and methodological questions and concerns led me to adopt the 'bricoleur' stance as researcher, while conducting fieldwork in an emergency department, a cardiothoracic unit, a hospice and the community. Denzin and Lincoln (1994, p.3) argued that the qualitative researcher's role is like that of the bricoleur, namely someone who brings elements of texts, images, representations, interpretations and phenomena together to form a bricolage: this is akin to a collage. The bricoleur is someone who uses instruments and tools for purposes for which they may not have been designed, and 'gets the job done' according to the tools at hand and what is needed at the time (see Gobbi, 2005; Weinstein and Weinstein, 1991).

This approach can illuminate the daily practices of learning in the workplace and enable the 'tacit' aspects of learning that are driven by the learner to be revealed in new ways. In other words, the chapter argues that the bricoleur approach can enable us to explore aspects of the 'hidden curricula' learning, in the 'messy' workplace of nursing. There are two core ideas associated with this: first, how one investigates the tacit, intuition and knowing-in-action; second, how to deal with the possibility that they may not exist as unique phenomena. However, a word of caution: it is impossible in a single chapter to offer an extensive summary of these concepts, so I shall restrict the debates to issues related to the conduct of research related to learning in practice. For the sake of brevity,

I will use the abbreviation TIRA to represent the study of the tacit, intuition and reflection-/knowing-in-action. As is discussed later, these terms are often confused in the literature.

The implications of studying TIRA: the definition dilemmas
. . . .

Each of the TIRA concepts is contested, and a full debate is beyond the remit of this chapter. Lumby (1991) suggested that intuition, reflection, thinking and knowing-in-action are at least equivalent terms, if not synonymous, while others questioned their very existence. Within the literature, the terms are sometimes used interchangeably, causing confusion, but, more important, the definitions relate to the disciplinary perspective of the author, whether philosophical, theological, psychological or feminist, for example. Let us commence with an analysis of the tacit. Polanyi (1966) classically described the tacit as a form of human knowing where we can 'know more than we can tell' (p.4). He proposed that the tacit is a form of human knowledge that emerges from a 'harmonious view of thought and existence, rooted in the universe' (p.4), albeit constrained by a cognitive discourse – no doubt a consequence of his own situatedness within a scientific and philosophical community of the 1950s and 1960s. For Polanyi (1958), the personal participation of the knower is essential in all acts of understanding. Knowing is a skilful action requiring an active comprehension of the known (p.vii). It may require effort, attention, indwelling and the establishment of a meaningful relationship between previous experience and the present. Indwelling is the interplay between the focal and subsidiary awareness (concepts outlined shortly). This relationship incorporates 'shaping or integrating tacit power by which all knowledge is discovered and, once discovered; is held to be true' (Polanyi, 1966, p.6). Note the 'orienting' and searching nature of the tacit and its association with discovering knowledge, discerning its veracity and acting with intentions.

Polanyi's explanation, and discussion, of two kinds of mutually exclusive knowing within the tacit (the focal and the subsidiary), offer a partial explanation for the problematic of the 'unsayable' aspects that are associated with these concepts. The focal is that to which we focus our attention, while the subsidiary is that which is subsumed within the total awareness. Thus, when focusing on the adjustment of an intravenous drip rate, I have a subsidiary awareness of the feel of the switch in my hand. In moving my attention to the switch, I lose focus on the drops. Polanyi suggests that objects held in subsidiary awareness, like an external tool, may become an extension of self, enabling the person to achieve or signify something (1958, p.61). Thus, 'we know the first term only by relying on our awareness of it for attending to the second' (1966, p.10). Similarly, it is possible that the nurse, in focusing on the patient, may not recognise the tacit knowing which is employed in so doing, where: 'Our conceptual imagination, like its artistic counterpart, draws inspiration from contact with experience' (1958, p.46). This interface/interaction between experience and the conceptual imagination is no doubt a potential component of the practitioner's ability to generate something new, but also mirrors the impact of the mind/body discourse split. In other words, new ideas, innovations and concepts can emerge from this interaction between the concrete experience and the imagination: the 'I wonder if?' moments in daily practice.

The other dilemma in trying to think in words or articulate what we know, is how we overcome the problems that arise from the dualism issue mentioned previously. For example, in Western languages and societies, we tend to polarise nouns and concepts into two components, e.g. positive/negative, subject/object, insider/outsider and so forth. It is difficult to express in words items, or concepts, that are neither solely an object nor a subject. For example, think about the way we struggle in English because we do not have a neutral expression for a person. To avoid gender bias by using he or she, we resort to s/he or the plural form 'their'. Similarly, people sometimes find it difficult to express those concepts that are at the heart of the clinical relationship between the client and the professional, where the client and practitioner know each other. Two concepts or images from Polanyi (1958, p.65) are particularly relevant here – namely, what he calls the 'act of hope', and 'striving to fulfil an obligation'. Polanyi likens this commitment to *love*. This sense of commitment may be directed towards a person (client) or thing (a pressure sore). For example, the commitment may direct action towards another person who could be a patient, relative, oneself, colleague, or towards theories or beliefs, the profession, institutions or organisations. This commitment influences our actions and our thoughts.

Polanyi also debates the transmission of skilful actions from one person to another. Polanyi states that skilful performance (here referring to the art of 'doing') is achieved by adhering to rules that are not known as such to the performers. While they may know the 'rules of art', these rules can only guide them if they are 'integrated into the practical knowledge of the art' (1958, p.50). However, until the art can be specified in detail, it cannot be transmitted by pre-scription, only by 'example from master to apprentice' through tradition. In such transmission, the apprentice has to submit to authority, placing trust in the master and emulating his practices. The analogy with nursing is apt, especially when the art is 'essentially inarticulate'. Dreyfus and Dreyfus (1986) draw on Polanyi's work, discussing the need to 'Decide in which areas it [nursing] can tolerate mere competence and in which areas it wishes to practice old fashioned training and apprenticeship so as to preserve old fashioned expertise' (p.188).

However, where the transmission of knowledge involves what I have called the 'little secrets' of practice (Gobbi, 1998, p.197) and is within a strong oral culture, then Polanyi's (1966) conclusion that 'the transmission of knowledge from one generation to another must be predominantly tacit' has profound implications for the development of practitioners (p.61). To Polanyi (1958), connoisseurship, an art of knowing, like skilful performance, 'can be communicated only by example, not by precept' (p.54). Connoisseurship is the discernment acquired from extensive practice and training, rather than the systematic acquisition of knowledge. Interestingly, one of Polanyi's examples of connoisseurship is that of the physician recognising heart sounds. In describing the personal knowing of the physician, Polanyi overlooks the necessary requirement to be a skilful performer in the *use* of the stethoscope. Drawing on Polanyi, then, the skilful performer is one who sets personal standards that the self evaluates, while the connoisseur values entities through standards that he has set 'for their excellence'. Polanyi considers that through the personal 'coefficient' (p.312), the commitment to universal standards transcends the individual's subjectivity and thus 'bridges 'the disjunction between subjectivity and objectivity' (p.300).

An examination of Polanyi's work indicates several dimensions of the tacit and skilful acts of knowing and doing:

- The tacit contains inarticulate and unspecifiable elements.
- Examination of these inarticulate and unspecifiable elements may be possible.
- Where skill is predominantly tacit, it requires transmission from master to apprentice.
- Awareness may be focal or subsidiary.
- Concepts like 'hope', 'commitment', 'obligation' and 'responsibility' are associated with personal knowing.
- Skilfulness and connoisseurship may involve 'indwelling' and different evaluative components.

Following on from our study of the tacit or personal knowing, we can now turn to intuition and reflection-in-action. These concepts are often associated with the tacit. As Bastick (1982) argued, there are no precise definitions of intuition, but rather there tend to be descriptions of what he termed 20 associated properties, including emotional involvement, subjective certainty of correctness, empathy and kinaesthetic knowledge of the Other. Within the nursing tradition, researchers like Benner (1994) have assumed that intuition existed, defining it as 'understanding without rationale' (Benner and Tanner, 1987), or in the words of Schraeder and Fischer (1987): 'The sudden inexplicable feeling that something is wrong, even if medical tests cannot confirm the patient's altered state' (p.47).

Intriguingly, from a philosophical perspective, Rorty (1967) defined intuition as 'immediate apprehension', where apprehension refers to disparate states like sensation, knowledge and mystical rapport. Furthermore, Rorty (1967) noted distinct differences among terms the hunch, the 'immediate knowledge of the truth' and knowledge of a concept. The hunch is 'unjustified true belief not preceded by inference'; 'immediate knowledge' of a truth refers to knowledge not preceded by inference and does not refer to a temporal concept; and 'knowledge of a concept' refers to occasions when knowledge is not accompanied by an ability to define it. Another perspective is a 'non-propositional' knowledge of an entity. Here, although knowledge is a necessary condition for the intuition of the entity, it may be sense perceptions, intuitions about universals and mystical or inexpressible intuitions. Rorty's use of the word 'immediate' is in stark contrast to the nursing literature. For example, for Rorty there is no association with time passing, whereas nursing writers like Paul and Heaslip (1995) construct 'immediate' to refer to 'sudden in onset/time'. Recently, however, reference to the perspectives of other disciplines is more common. For further detail on intuition in nursing, see King and Appleton (1997) and Rew and Barrow (2007).

Another descriptor ascribed to intuition is that it is synonymous with 'know-how': the 'understanding that effortlessly occurs upon seeing similarities with previous experience' (Dreyfus and Dreyfus, 1986). From this perspective, intuition is the product of deep situational involvement and recognition of similarity, and as an 'everyday' experience, it implies a 'sameness', a 'reproducible' nature or a 'commonness'.

Gender links and attributions between women and intuition were noted as early as 1987, when Rew and Barrow articulated the concern that the use of intuition by women, particularly in nursing practice, had been 'ignored, denigrated or denied', thus eliciting a quite different response to the 'insights' or 'intuitive leaps' described in the more male-dominated fields of mathematics and science. In these fields, intuitive leaps were not only well documented but also seemingly integral to the stages of creativity, e.g. scientists like Einstein (Wertheimer, 1961). In the works of Benner (1984), Watson (1985), Meleis (1991) and Street

(1992), there emerged an increasing (or regained) legitimacy accorded to intuition and subjective knowing. Paterson and Zderad (1976) advocated integrated approaches, arguing that the ability to combine intuition and analysis is nursing's methodology, being both subjective and objective. In a similar way, Pyles and Stern (1983) proposed a nursing 'Gestalt': 'a synergy of logic and intuition involving both conceptual and sensory acts' related to timing, accessibility and an effective mentoring relationship. This notion of synergy also emerged from the work of McCutcheon and Pincombe (2001), who found that nine categories were associated with intuition and that the summative effect, or synergy, was greater than the individual effects.

Shotter, in his analysis of Vico (1993, p.54), proposed that intuition may be an aspect of the *sensus communis* (common sense) in which 'feelings or intuition' have an established 'something' with common significance. According to Shotter, Vico's *sensus communis* arises from socially shared identities of feelings in which an experience, event or circumstance has generated a shared sense with a subsequent 'imaginative universal'. Vico's use of the phrase 'feelings or intuitions' is itself significant, indicating that perhaps:

● feelings are intuitions
● feelings are not intuitions but, rather, intuitions are an alternative to feeling
● the word intuition is the imaginative universal.

The philosophical challenge presented by 'feelings' is well debated by Langer (1967), who noted that the effects caused by feelings are physically describable, yet the feeling of them is not. Langer contended that feelings are fundamental to the act of knowing. This argument links the cognition, its accompanying 'feeling' component and the behaviours that may be consequent to the 'intuition'. Bastick (1982) argued the importance of intuition to learning when he claimed that 'intuitions are basic to the educational process' (p.100). If we accept that feelings and intuition are essential to the act of knowing, then as educators our challenge is to understand how intuition is learnt, how it can be developed, and whether it is characteristically different between the novice and the expert.

Learning to be intuitive: intuition in the naïve/ novice and expert

The role and existence of intuition in the novice is another disputed issue, based largely upon arguments concerning the presence or absence of an a priori experience of knowledge and whether it is the product of personal involvement in a certain practical or theoretical activity. DiSessa (1983), writing in the context of learning physics, proposed that intuition (as p-prims, or phenomenological primitives) changes from having an explanatory effect with the novice to a heuristic outcome for the expert. P-prims are naïve concepts or general principles that guide actions unconsciously. The novice needs to learn which of these principles are 'real', important, or inappropriate and which, therefore, need to be discarded. Experts, having learnt how to evaluate these concepts, can use them in their decision-making processes. Similarly, in the nursing context, expert nurses argued that the deliberation required to analyse intuitive decisions or processes no longer makes them 'intuitive' (Orme and Maggs, 1993). Benner (1984) attributed intuition to expertise, whereas Ruth-Sahd (1993) argued that the novice has intuitive aspects through 'knowing the person'. Several researchers have discussed the connections among 'intuition', risk taking, conviction, confidence and knowing in the neonatal environment (Benner *et al.*, 1996; Orme and Maggs, 1993; Jenny and Logan, 1992). With respect to student nurses, King and Appleton (1997) argued that intuition occurs '[i]n response to knowledge, is a trigger for nursing action and/or reflection and thus has a direct bearing on analytical processes in patient/client care' (p.201). Here, we can see that intuition is associated not only with the concepts of trying to do something and acting intentionally but also with 'knowing-in-action' (what and how to do) and the interchangeable concepts of thinking-in-action and reflecting-in-action. First, let us consider further the issue of learning to try before focusing on our last concepts associated with knowing-in-action.

Shotter (1975) discussed how individuals learn how to try in a manner that makes sense to others and, citing Dreyfus (1967), he reminded us that the process of trying enables one to know how to try. He described how persons come to *act intentionally* (p.110) when their actions are informed by 'their knowledge of what they are acting on' and that persons can 'come to act intending meanings' (ibid) in their action. He argued that the person is 'faced' with the challenge of acting intelligibly and responsibly rather than just intelligently. Beckett (1995) echoed this dimension of acting *towards* an outcome when he debated the extent to which reflection endorses rational action. Beckett's conclusion was that there is no such thing as Schön's (1983) reflection-in-action. At the sub-episodic level, there is judgement, which is associated with trying toward achievement and is accompanied by a series of actions. While there is dynamism between the episodic and the sub-episodic, it is not reflective; rather, it is reflexive. In other words, intentions are mediated by other beliefs and contexts, and to paraphrase

Shotter (1975, p.91), human action is constructed by the interplay between the individual's attempt to realise their 'projects, goals, enterprises or ideals'. This insight has particular relevance when considering the impact of responsibility upon the learning of the practitioner, whose 'projects, goals, enterprises or ideals' may be specifically related to a client or family.

It is important to acknowledge that reflection-in-action implies two activities, knowing and doing, which are conceived of as being different yet connected. Eraut (1994) first noted the difficulty in defining reflection-in-action because Schön, the major proponent, did not use sustained argument but, rather, employed metaphor and example. Schön (1987, 1983) argued for a model of professional practice in which the 'artistry, intuitive and creative' dimensions of practice were valued. Schön (1983) described knowing-in-action as the 'characteristic mode of ordinary practical knowledge' while 'reflecting-in-action' referred to the common sense notion that 'we can think about doing something while doing it' (p.54). During this process, the practitioner may evolve a way of doing it. Reflection-in-action is considered to 'hinge on the experience of surprise' (p.57); and to 'act as a corrective to overlearning', thereby enabling one to 'make sense of uncertain situations' (p.61); it involves a form of action research, and is coached rather than taught. Reflection-in-action can be seen in the performance of practitioners who demonstrate 'professional artistry'. However, the paradox is that if an 'expert' increasingly acts through 'knowing in action' and is 'not surprised', then presumably s/he reflects *less* in action. Schön goes so far as to equate this with boredom, rigidity and a deteriorated service to the client group.

Schön's views on thinking/reflecting and knowing-in-action were influenced by Polanyi's work. Both Schön and Polanyi referred to the somewhat 'ordinary' nature of thinking while doing, and stated clearly that the *knowing is in the action*. In other words, knowing is part of action. Reflection upon a previous episode of knowing something is often accompanied by reflection (thinking) in the present and the emergence of what Schön (1991) subsequently described as a 'reflective conversation' with the matters in hand. In other words people are having their own internal dialogue with the previous episode of knowing and their knowing or thoughts in current moment and situation. Beckett (1995) described Schön's reflection-in-action as the 'hot and immediate slice of practice within which the professional can make a difference then and there' (p.104). He analysed 'time' within the slice (or episode) of practice, and he argued that the practitioner seeks to achieve that which is 'right' and consequently that which is providential. He pointed out that reflection-in-action is problematic because it is difficult to:

> conceptualise an epistemology of occurent action which leaves the power of human purposes intact. We act because we *want* (that is desire) to. But we also act because we *have* to. (p.114)

Like Eraut, Beckett questioned aspects of Schön's concept, especially the phenomenon known as 'reflection-in-action'. Beckett demonstrated his criticisms through reference to two points: first, through analysis of trying/anticipation, and second, through references to intentionality. Greenwood (1993), Lauder (1994) and Beckett (1995) challenged Schön's conception of reflection-in-action, arguing that Aristotle's practical syllogism and practical wisdom might be more apt, a claim supported by Benner *et al.* (1996). The argument here is that Schön assumed that thinking occurs before action and separated thinking from action. Aristotle's practical wisdom referred to a form of knowledge (knowing) that is primarily concerned with the knowledge required to do good for another person, involving the effective and moral way of doing so. Practical syllogism involves the consideration of the ways of doing something in practice and the consequences of that action. Thus nursing knowledge and deliberative knowing-in-action (in its broadest sense) are focused on the knowledge, effective ways and means to do good for another, having taken account of the moral implications and consequences of acting (or not acting). These theoretical discussions inform the discussion of fieldwork in the second part of this chapter, which sets out to explore with practitioners what they knew, felt and thought during nursing activities.

Investigating the tacit, intuitive and knowing-in-action

The methodological 'headaches' associated with investigating the tacit are well known. Simply, how does one 'find out' what is happening or being experienced when a person reveals, or appears to be using, intuition, reflection or thinking-in-action (whatever they may be!)? Two methods can seem obvious: observation and engaging in 'talk about the phenomenon'. Meerabeau (1992), Benner (1984) and Benner *et al.* (1996) argued that verbal methods alone are insufficient because practitioners create new knowledge that is not coded or published. Retrospective accounts are not without their flaws concerning authenticity, post hoc rationality, incomplete memory and tendencies to reconstruct events. The use of 'think aloud' techniques was considered for this research, but rejected on two grounds.

First, it is difficult, and perhaps in some instances unethical to do this in actual clinical practice. Second, it is not without its methodological flaws (see Ericsson and Simon's (1998) classic text). Dreyfus (1982) emphasised the importance of the individual's account rather than the observer's, although careful observation when someone undergoes 'real world learning' has its place. Steier (1991) argued that patterns of unknowing may get 'unconcealed in conversation' and that stories may reveal 'social ways of seeing and doing' (p.167). This indicated that attending to the conversations, accounts and narratives as well as observing practitioners might enable me to elicit their 'ways of seeing, knowing and doing' nursing through their discourse. Both Polanyi (1958) and Polkinghorne (1992) considered that the analysis of narrative could reveal, at a cultural level, shared beliefs and the transmission of values (see Chapter 10 for treatment of narrative research approaches). It seems sensible, therefore, to consider that the 'tacit or intuitive' and any 'thinking or reflecting-in-action' can be identified by analysing practitioner activities, discourses and 'talk' about what they are thinking, what they know and what they are doing. Those who argue that there are connections among discourse, knowledge and expertise support this position; for example, Foucault (1973, 1972), Fairclough (1992a, 1992b), Benner (1984) and Benner *et al.* (1996).

I set out to engage in longitudinal intermittent participant observations with three individuals at different stages of development and in three different contexts (*see* Table 6.1). As you can see, I chose to work in areas in which I was familiar, a stranger, an expert and just competent. Therefore, I was able to be a subject of the research myself, using my own experiences as a participant observer and noticing the extent to which I learnt, thought and experienced during the clinical contexts of the research. I adopted the role of 'companion' registered nurse, acting as if 'I was an agency nurse'.

The research involved collecting data relating to:
- direct and participant observation in the tradition of Gold (1958) and Becker (1969); this meant that the researcher (myself) participated in the daily lives of the group, individuals or situation under study and contrasted their experiences with her observations
- the researcher's immediate and recalled experience, thoughts, feelings and behaviours
- the participant's immediate and recalled experience, thoughts, feelings and behaviours
- pertinent knowledge/knowings from other 'informants' in the field

- material gleaned from tape recordings, accounts of commentaries, interviews
- analysis of pertinent documents.

It was important to consider what Polkinghorne (1992) outlined as the connections and relationships between an individual's perceptions, and to determine whether they are:

- the same as, or not
- are similar or dissimilar
- are an instance of
- stand for something (i.e. an icon, index or symbol)
- are a part of
- are a cause of …

TABLE 6.1 Participants

Participant	Duration of observation	Clinical context	Participant's degree of expertise	My degree of expertise
A	18 months with follow-up interviews at 24 and 36 months	Cardiothoracic	Newly qualified	Expert clinical background
B	8 months	Emergency nursing	Expert	Related critical care experience but active in emergency since a student
C	18 months	Hospice care to community palliative care	Experienced, becoming expert	No prior experience in these contexts; general skills only – stranger

Analysing the data assumes that the researcher can recognise and identify the subject matter, reminding us of Meno's dilemma. However, by being present in the field I hoped to capture the attributed 'instances of' the tacit and intuition and then determine or explore any connections with other similar episodes or accounts. While there is no universal agreement about the factors associated with alleged intuitive episodes, participant observation provided the opportunity to capture them, should they exist, as near as possible to the event. Aside from claiming that the study was informed by ethnography and hermeneutic in approach, the decision-making concerning the fieldwork was pragmatic.

The methodology had to deal with a variety of epistemological (ways of knowing) and ontological (ways of being) positions derived from an array of philosophical and disciplinary backgrounds, e.g. psychology, sociology, science and linguistics. The second major challenge was to determine how to handle the data. Analysing accounts and 'accounts of accounts' naturally means dealing with 'text and talk' and consideration of discourse analysis (DA), particularly as ethnographic accounts culminate in texts. An issue is whether DA is sufficiently rigorous to deal with an interpersonal activity like nursing that incorporates knowing of a person with a moral significance and knowing of the case (Steedman, 1991). Another important dimension is the recognition that what we know/experience cannot always be captured in words or speech.

As you can see, like Levi-Strauss's bricoleur (1966), I was already drawing on 'bits and pieces' from a variety of traditions, and this was to be replicated in the process of data analysis, when I drew on elements of DA to help me interpret and 'read' the experience of the participants as well as to 'read' and interpret the written text.

Handling the data, becoming a bricoleur

Before proceeding further, it is timely to consider the concept of the bricoleur as researcher. The term was first ascribed to Levi-Strauss (1966), when he explored whether thoughts or actions could be distinguished as scientific or mythical. The word subsequently referred to someone who 'works with his hands and uses devious means compared to those of the craftsman … a Jack of all trades or a kind of professional do-it-yourself man' (Levi-Strauss 1966, pp.16–17). Levi-Strauss stressed that the 'Jack of all trades' person is of better standing than the English 'odd-job man'. In other words, as I shall demonstrate, a bricoleur selects and adapts research methods and tools according to the research needs, rather than for the purpose or discipline for which they may have been designed originally. While Morse (1991) warned that researchers adopting this approach could create a sloppy 'mishmash', more recently this has become part of a movement towards 'guerrilla theorising' of practitioner theory (Reid, 2008). As we shall see, I concur with Reid, who argued that the related concepts of bricoleur, improvisation and abduction provide a beginning infrastructure for practice-based theory development. Reid explained abduction as the process of formulating plausible explanations from empirical observations and other knowledge sources.

Data analysis became predicated upon the acknowledgement that experience can be read as if it were text (see Usher, 1992a); that account should be taken of all the senses, feelings and knowing associated with nursing activity and clinical knowing; and that observation of individuals over time should also reveal the range of their knowing, but, in addition, record their learning and development. The product of participant observation in this instance was also text, so again DA had the potential to assist in the analysis of key sections of data. In this respect:

- the study *was* hermeneutical because it defined text as 'any written or spoken product of (D) discourses'
- from an intentional perspective, I used both participant observation and DA as tools, rather than method
- the study was not an ethnography in the 'disciplinary' sense outlined by Hammersley (1992)
- the study assimilated material from other discourses rather than from a single defined discourse perspective
- in 'the grey' of researching, the normal and historically advocated role, expressions and forms of engagement could be transgressed
- while researching as bricoleur, I developed an analytical perspective that might 'mirror' aspects of the nursing context.

O'Collins and Farrugia (1991) described hermeneutics as the theory and practice of understanding and interpreting texts, biblical or otherwise. In the attempt to understand and interpret, hermeneutics seeks to locate texts within their historical, situated context, striving to convey the 'meaning' to contemporary society (*see* Chapter 10). In so doing, hermeneutics recognises that a text 'can contain and convey meaning beyond the original author's explicit intention' (O'Collins and Farrugia, 1991, p.90). Inevitably, the role of the interpreter (translator or reader) is pivotal. The metaphor of the dialogue has been used to describe the conversational relationship between the interpreter, the text and by inference the original author(s). This dialogic nature of hermeneutics, the 'hermeneutical circle', arises from the works of theorists like Heidegger (1962) and Gadamer (1993). Furthermore, by considering experience as text (Usher, 1992b), the hermeneutical dimension may be applied to the reading of experience, as well as the reading of texts in a literal sense. 'Reading' is thus a metaphor of action. Table 6.2 demonstrates how I appropriated insights from various authors to help me analyse the data.

These next fieldwork examples illustrate the various uses of different strands of DA to handle the data. The first example is rooted in Austin's (1962) work concerning the performative and constative nature of sentences, that is sentences

TABLE 6.2 Analytical influences

Point	Influence	Source
1	(D) discourse can be both 'text and talk' and studied as topic and resource	Potter and Wetherell, 1987; Gilbert and Mulkay, 1984
2	DA is not restricted to the cognitive dimension; it can be plurisensorial	Woolgar, 1988; Gilbert and Mulkay, 1984
3	Sample size is determined by the process rather than inherently valuable for its size	Potter and Wetherell, 1987; Gilbert and Mulkay, 1984
4	Accounts of lived experience may include the four existentials of lived time, space, body and relation	Van Maanen, 1988
5	There may be interpretive variability generated by context; action and belief held by the participants	Gilbert and Mulkay, 1984
6	Potentially different repertoires may be encountered	Gilbert and Mulkay, 1984
7	The possible existence of 'collective consensus'	Gilbert and Mulkay, 1984; Gadamer, 1993
8	To consider evidence of changes in discourse/ knowledge and to consider whether particular classes of discourse may have precedence, or be stages in practitioner development	Gilbert and Mulkay, 1984
9	Texts may be evaluated in respect to their doing component, their descriptive element and the potential conventions associated with them, i.e. seeking the action orientation	Austin, 1962 (cited in Potter and Wetherell, 1987)
10	There may be indicators of accountability, responsibility and their attribution	Edwards and Potter, 1992
11	Consider the portrayal of fact and interest	Edwards and Potter, 1992
12	Explore links between the mode of action and the mode of representation and pertinent issues which arise in respect of the language functions of 'identity', 'relationships' and knowledgeing/ believing	Fairclough, 1992a
13	Consider the simultaneity of the present in relation to the simultaneity of the past	Foucault, 1972
14	Attend to the possibilities of 'silent murmurings' and 'intertextual' threads, the 'not said' and 'unsayable'	Foucault, 1972
15	Recognise the import of power/knowledge influences, but not at the expense of ignoring hegemonic, reciprocal or covenant relationships, i.e. consider the nature of the relationship	Bradshaw, 1994; Schluter and Lee, 1993; Foucault, 1972
16	Acknowledge how persons are recognised, positioned and relate to each other	Schluter and Lee, 1993; Foucault, 1972

may have a doing (performative) component and a descriptive element (revealing the current situation), with conventions associated with the words uttered and the related social activity. Practitioner A is describing a challenging incident from practice when she describes a patient thus:

> He's apyrexial, but I don't know if that is the paracetamol. I don't know if they are aware of that. There's something I can't put my finger on about that man. (A, month 11)

In the first sentence, A is stating a fact (he's apyrexial), and speculating (is the absence of a recordable fever due to the paracetamol?). She then wonders whether the medical staff may not be aware of that. Next, she indicates worry and an acknowledgement that there is something else to know, but she doesn't know what that might be. Her worry leads her to take subsequent action, with the spoken expression of worry, having what Austin calls a performative function. Her statement also acts as a signifier to others, drawing their attention to her concern that 'something' else may be happening.

Evidence of changing perspectives through the discourses was evidenced in the fieldwork, enabling me to chart A's learning and development (see her discourse and Gilbert and Mulkay, 1984). Her discourse patterns changed to the extent that when she reviewed a transcript of an interview from month 3 concerning a 'horrendous' event, A remarked spontaneously:

> Yes, I was going to say that to you Mary, the way I am talking even is different, the way it comes across as well isn't it?

And then:

> Yes, yes (.) and maybe even <u>NOW</u> 'horrendous episodes' I probably (.) I wouldn't find them so horrendous now. And becoming more attuned (.) to everything, (.) It concerns me that I used to see them as horrendous episodes [said with irony]. I think as well (.) because (.) if you regard them as horrendous episodes then I would say that you probably don't act as well as you may do. (A, month 15)
>
> (The transcript convention is from Jefferson, 1985).

In this next example, from work with C, I drew on Edwards and Potter (1992), who pointed out that activities occur in a sequence, in which psychological concepts such as reward, compliment, blame, invitation and responsibility reside. Furthermore, like Sampson (1993), they recognise the 'intertextual collective' other(s), in other words, the other people who are hidden, or referred to, within the text. This fieldwork example from observation work in a hospice refers to F, aged 17, whose grandmother, 'nan', is dying of cancer. C, the registered nurse I was observing, was conversing with her in a secluded sitting room. The example refers to 'others' who are silently present: the grandmother 'nan', F's parents, the 'other lady who had died' and myself:

> F wanted to know how quickly the end may come. C described the fact that for most people there was a warning signal … At this point C commented upon people 'going yellow' and wheezing. This in fact transpired to be the yellow colour of her nan, which C explained was due to her liver [disease]. The wheeziness was what F had observed from the other patient who had died. C managed to respond to these enquiries and seemed to be able to locate the contexts. This was one where I couldn't locate the context because I hadn't seen the other lady who had died. (notes with C, month 6)

While this extract describes an aspect of 'everyday life' of the staff in the hospice – namely, responding to the needs of relatives who have questions to ask – it is followed by C's account of the activities that were taking place during the interaction. C describes the situation thus:

> F alternatively looked at the two of us. I found myself actively trying to work out where to put my eyes, sometimes she would look at me and I would avoid F by looking at C, or I would smile and reinforce what was happening, or just nod. It was an intriguing position and as the observer, my presence was automatically becoming involved in the 'between us', I could not 'fade'. I could actively retreat, affirm, be still, or focus on them differently. I noticed that I seemed to be naturally emulating C's postures quite significantly. (Notes with C, month 6)

This extract illustrates how important it is to incorporate the intensity of this action as represented in the recalled account, and draws theoretically on the works of Foucault (1973), Bradshaw (1994) and Schluter and Lee (1993). These extracts demonstrate the pragmatic, embodied knowing/sensing of everyday practice. From the research perspective, I was using 'bits and pieces' to deal with specific aspects of the text, having drawn upon a range of authors from different traditions and contexts. This is the essence of researching as a bricoleur who views nursing as an 'embodied, bricoleur practice where practitioners draw on the "shards and fragments" of the situation-at-hand to resolve the needs of the individual patient for whom they care' (Gobbi, 2005, p.117).

As I have argued elsewhere (Gobbi, 2009, 2005), nursing's methodology draws on several scientific, artistic and social science traditions in the endeavour to care for the patient/client. It is pragmatic, strategic and concerned with Polanyi's personal commitment of the knower, the act of hope, striving to fulfil an obligation and the desire to improve the health and well being of another. To investigate the knowing of the practitioner, and to elicit the tacit, we need to cross the traditional disciplinary boundaries to find ways of revealing it. This means analysing the embodied, considering the purpose and meanings of utterances – not just their literal impact – and attending to that which is not said, as well as that found in verbalised communications.

Conclusion: workplace learning

There are several implications of TIRA and guerrilla theories for workplace learning. First, learning in the healthcare workplace is concerned with learning in action for action with people and relies upon a tacit pedagogy of searching for future or concurrent action to resolve the situations at hand (Gobbi, 2005, 1998). When the practice of the learner involves bricoleur activity, then it means that learners need to be helped to develop skills of imagination and improvisation, and to be open to new possibilities that can arise from the adoption, adaptation or reconstruction of existing theory, tools and practices. This is risky business, and may appear challenging in governance-driven, defensive practices. In these situations, learners need support from traditional methods like coaching and mentoring. Their learning will be shaped and determined by slippery issues of 'hope and commitment', by the articulation and transmission of practices without substantive empirical 'legitimised' evidence. Learners are faced with competing messages and paradigms, evidence-based practice versus the 'little secrets' of practitioner-based knowing passed ritualistically, with or without reasonable explanation. Clinical educators need to reflect carefully on their practices and identify their own personal knowing so that they can reveal it to the learner. Certainly the science and artistry of practice and theoretical knowing should be acquired and promulgated, but so too should the mysterious world of the tacit, intuitive and knowing-as-action in the daily practice of the bricoleur.

References

Austin, J. (1962) *How to Do Things with Words.* London, Oxford University Press.

Bastick, T. (1982) *Intuition: how we think and act.* Chichester, John Wiley & Sons.

Becker, H. S. (1969) Problems in the publication of field studies. In: G. J. McCall and J. L. Simmons (eds) (1969) *Issues in Participant Observation: a text and reader.* London, Addison Wesley.

Beckett, D. (1995) *Adult Education as Professional Practice.* Unpublished doctor of philosophy thesis. Sydney, University of Technology.

Benner, P. (1984) *From Novice to Expert.* Menlo Park, CA, Addison-Wesley.

Benner, P. (ed.) (1994) *Interpretive Phenomenology: embodiment, caring, and ethics in health and illness.* London, Sage.

Benner, P. and Tanner, C. (1987) Clinical judgment: how expert nurses use intuition. *American Journal of Nursing,* 87(1), 23–31.

Benner, P. A., Tanner, C. A. and Chesla, C. A. (1996) *Expertise in Nursing Practice: caring, clinical judgment, and ethics.* New York, NY, Springer.

Bradshaw, A. (1994) *Lighting the Lamp: the spiritual dimension of nursing care.* London, Scutari.

Denzin, N. K. and Lincoln, Y. S. (eds) (1994) *Handbook of Qualitative Research.* London, Sage.

DiSessa, A. A. (1983) Phenomenology and the evolution of intuition. In: D. Gentner and A. Stevens (1983) *Mental Models.* Hillsdale, NJ, Lawrence Erlbaum Associates, pp.15–33.

Dreyfus, H. L. (1967) Why computers must have bodies in order to be intelligent. *Review of Metaphysics,* 21(1), 13–32.

Dreyfus, H. L. and Dreyfus, S. E. (1986) *Mind over Machine: the power of human intuition and expertise in the era of the computer.* New York, The Free Press.

Dreyfus, S. E. (1982) Formal models vs human situational understanding: inherent limitations on the modelling of business expertise. *Office: Technology and People,* 1, 133–65.

Edwards, D. and Potter, J. (1992) *Discursive Psychology.* London, Sage.

Eraut, M. (1994) *Developing Professional Knowledge and Competence.* London, Falmer Press.

Ericsson, K. A. and Simon, H. A. (1998) How to study thinking in everyday life: contrasting think-aloud protocols with descriptions and explanations of thinking. *Mind, Culture, and Activity,* 5(3), 178–86.

Fairclough, N. (1992a) *Discourse and Social Change.* Oxford, Polity Press.

Fairclough, N. (ed.) (1992b) *Critical Language Awareness.* London, Longman.

Foucault, M. (1972) *The Archaeology of Knowledge,* trans. A. M. Sheridan Smith. London, Routledge.

Foucault, M. (1973) *The Birth of the Clinic: an archaeology of medical perception,* trans. A. M. Sheridan Smith. London, Routledge.

Gadamer, H. G. (1993) *Truth and Method,* trans. J. Weinsheimer and D. G. Marshall. 2nd rev. edn. London, Shead & Ward.

Gilbert, G. and Mulkay, M. (1984) *Opening Pandora's Box: a sociological analysis of scientist's discourse*. Cambridge, Cambridge University Press.

Gobbi, M. (1998) *Searching for Intuition: discovering the unsayable within discourses of nursing practice*. Unpublished doctoral thesis. University of Southampton, Faculty of Educational Studies.

Gobbi, M. (2005) Nursing practice as bricoleur activity: a concept explored. *Nursing Inquiry*, 12(2), 117–25.

Gobbi, M. (2009) Learning in the workplace community: the generation of professional capital. In: A. Le May (ed.) *Communities of Practice in Health and Social Care*. Chichester, Wiley-Blackwell, pp.66–82.

Gold, R. L. (1958) Roles in sociological field analysis. *Social Forces*, 36: 217–23.

Greenwood, J. (1993) Reflective practice: a critique of the work of Argyris and Schön. *Journal of Advanced Nursing*, 18(8), 1183–7.

Hammersley, M. (1992) *What's Wrong with Ethnography?* London, Routledge.

Heidegger, M. (1962) *Being and Time*, trans. J. Macquarrie and E. Robinson. Oxford, Blackwell.

Jefferson, G. (1985). An exercise in the transcription and analysis of laughter. In: T. A. van Dijk (ed.) *Handbook of Discourse Analysis, Vol. 3: discourse and dialogue*. London, Academic Press, pp.25–34.

Jenny, J. and Logan, J. (1992) Knowing the patient: one aspect of clinical knowledge. *Image: Journal of Nursing Scholarship*, 24(4), 254–8.

King, L. and Appleton, J. (1997) Intuition: a critical review of the research and rhetoric. *Journal of Advanced Nursing*, 26(1), 194–202.

Langer, S. K. (1967) *Mind: an essay in human feeling, vol. 1*. Baltimore MD, John Hopkins Press.

Lauder, W. (1994) Beyond reflection: practical wisdom and the practical syllogism. *Nurse Education Today*, 14(2), 91–8.

Levi-Strauss, C. (1966) *The Savage Mind*. London, Weidenfeld & Nicolson.

Lumby, J. (1991) Threads of an emerging discipline, praxis, reflection, rhetoric and research. In: G. Gray and R. Pratt (eds) *Towards a Discipline of Nursing*. Edinburgh, Churchill Livingstone, pp.461–84.

McCutcheon, H. H. I and Pincombe, J. (2001) Intuition: an important tool in the practice of nursing. *Journal of Advanced Nursing*, 35(3), 342–8.

Meerabeau, L. (1992) Tacit nursing knowledge: an untapped resource or a methodological headache? *Journal of Advanced Nursing*, 17(1), 108–12.

Meleis, A. I. (1991) *Theoretical Nursing: development and progress*. 2nd edn. New York, NY, Lippincott.

Morse, J. (ed.) (1991) *Qualitative Nursing Research: a contemporary dialogue*. Rev. edn. London, Sage.

O'Collins, G. and Farrugia, E. G. (1991). *A Concise Dictionary of Theology*. London, Harper Collins.

Orme, L. and Maggs, C. (1993) Decision making in clinical practice: how do expert nurses, midwives and health visitors make decisions? *Nurse Education Today*, 13(4), 270–6.

Paterson, J. G. and Zderad, L. T. (1976) *Humanistic Nursing*. New York, NY, John Wiley & Sons.

Paul, R. W. and Heaslip, P. (1995) Critical thinking and intuitive nursing practice. *Journal of Advanced Nursing*, 22(1), 40–7.

Plato (1966) *Protagoras and Meno*, trans. W. K. C. Guthrie. Middlesex, Penguin.

Polanyi, M. (1958) *Personal Knowledge*. London, Routledge & Kegan Paul.

Polanyi, M. (1966) *The Tacit Dimension*. London, Routledge & Kegan Paul.

Polkinghorne, D. E. (1992) Post modern epistemology of practice. In: S. Kvale (ed.) *Psychology and Post Modernism*. London, Sage, pp.146–65.

Potter, H. and Wetherell, M. (1987) *Discourse and Social Psychology: beyond attitudes and behaviour*. London, Sage.

Pyles, S. H. and Stern, P. N. (1983) Discovery of nursing gestalt in critical care nursing: the importance of the gray gorilla syndrome. *Image: The Journal of Nursing Scholarship*, 15(2), 51–8.

Reid, P. G. (2008) Practitioner as theorist: a reprise: *Nursing Science Quarterly*, 21(4), 315–21.

Rew, L. and Barrow, E. M. (1987) Intuition: a neglected hallmark of nursing knowledge. *Advances in Nursing Science*, 10(1), 49–62.

Rew, L and Barrow E. M. (2007) State of the science: intuition in nursing, a generation of studying the phenomenon. *Advances in Nursing Science*, 30(1), e1–25.

Rorty, R. (1967) Intuition. In: P. Edwards (ed.) *The Encyclopaedia of Philosophy, Vol. 4*. London, Collier-MacMillan Limited, pp.204–12.

Ruth-Sahd, L. A. (1993) A modification of Benner's hierarchy of clinical practice: the development of clinical intuition in the novice trauma nurse. *Holistic Nursing Practice*, 7(3), 8–14.

Sampson, E. E. (1993) *Celebrating the Other: a dialogic account of human nature*. New York, NY, Harvester Wheatsheaf.

Schluter, M. and Lee, D (1993) *The R Factor*. London, Hodder & Stoughton.

Schön, D. A. (1983) *The Reflective Practitioner*. New York, NY, Basic Books.

Schön, D. A. (1987) *Educating the Reflective Practitioner*. San Francisco, CA, Jossey-Bass.

Schön, D. A. (ed.) (1991) *The Reflective Turn: case studies in and on educational practice*. New York, NY, Teachers College, Columbia University.

Schraeder, B. D. and Fischer, D. K. (1987) Using intuitive knowledge in the neonatal intensive care nursery. *Holistic Nursing Practice*, 1(3), 45–51.

Shotter, J. (1975) *Images of Man in Psychological Research*. London, Methuen & Co.

Shotter, J. (1993) *Conversational Realities: constructing life through language*. London, Sage.

Steedman, H. (1991) On the relations between seeing, interpreting and knowing. In: F. Steier (ed.) *Research and Reflexivity*. London, Sage, pp.53–62.

Steier, F. (ed.) (1991) *Research and Reflexivity*. London, Sage.

Street, A. F. (1992) *Inside Nursing: a critical ethnography of clinical nursing practice*. New York, State University of New York Press.

Usher, R. (1992a) Must we always research ourselves? Problems of writing and reflexivity in research. *Occasional Papers in Education and Interdisciplinary Studies*, 1, 9–16.

Usher, R. (1992b) Experience in adult education: a post-modern critique. *Journal of Philosophy of Education*, 1(2), 201–14.

Van Maanen, J. (1988) *Tales of the Field: on writing ethnography*. Chicago, IL, University of Chicago Press.

Watson, J. (1985) *Nursing: human science or human care*. St. Louis, MO, Mosby.

Weinstein, D. and Weinstein, N. A. (1991) Georg Simmel: sociological flâneur bricoleur. *Theory, Culture and Society*, 8(3), 151–68.

Wertheimer, M. (1961) *Productive Thinking*. London, Tavistock.

Woolgar, S. (ed.) (1988) *Knowledge and Reflexivity: new frontiers in the sociology of knowledge*. London, Sage.

7

Learning in the operating theatre

A social semiotic perspective

*Jeff Bezemer, Gunther Kress, Alexandra Cope
and Roger Kneebone*

Introduction

Learning has become a key issue across different disciplines. The school is no longer seen as the only significant site of learning, and learning is no longer seen as a matter of the 'mind' alone (Säljö, 2009; Lave and Wenger, 1991). The approach put forward in this chapter embraces these changes in the theorisation of learning. The starting points of our approach are, first, that teaching and learning are *social* practices. Hence our theory is a socially based theory, concerned with the interaction between people and the identities and social roles they take up across different sites, including clinical workplaces. Our second starting point is that teaching and learning are instances of *communication*, so that a theory of learning and teaching is set within the general frame of a theory of communication. We study communication not to identify 'communication failures' in clinical work (see Lingard *et al.*, 2004) but to draw attention to the resourcefulness of clinicians as communicators and the complexities of their encounters with patients and other clinicians, whether as teachers or as learners.

Our theory of communication – and by implication, of learning – is a social semiotic one. Its focus is *semiosis* – that is, how people 'make meaning'; how they make sense of what other people say and do, and what they themselves say and do 'to make things happen'. To help develop this theory further, and to address specific questions about *clinical* learning, we have analysed audio and video recordings of interactions in the operating theatres of a teaching hospital in London. We used a wireless microphone worn by one of the surgeons, and inbuilt video cameras, allowing us to capture those things to which surgeons typically orient themselves – that is, their hands, their instruments and the parts of the patient's body that they operate on. In addition to these recordings, we kept detailed field notes of all operations observed, particularly noting changes in the spatial configuration of participants around the operating table, and we made photographs of the screens, books and other media that are used in the operating theatre (see Bezemer *et al.*, 2011a for more methodological details).

Video recordings are indispensable for our social semiotic research, not least in clinical settings, since communication and learning are instantiated in the fine-grained detail of subtle body movements. For instance, in an operating theatre, surgeons' shifts in their direction of gaze from operative field to scrub nurse may suggest the onset of a request for an instrument. These shifts occur in split seconds. They cannot be captured on the spot and in field notes by researchers, let alone recalled in interviews by the research participants after the observed event. A video record allows us to begin to analyse these practices. Detailed analysis of video recordings of workplaces and educational settings is now well established in social research (Heath *et al.*, 2010; Kissmann, 2009), including social research in clinical settings (Iedema *et al.*, 2006). The theoretical and methodological assumptions underlying these studies vary somewhat. Most video-based studies of the operating theatre and its adjacent rooms, such as the anaesthetic room, are based in conversation analysis. These studies highlight the 'practical accomplishment' of clinical work (Bezemer *et al.*, 2011b; Koschmann *et al.*, 2011; Svensson *et al.*, 2007; Mondada, 2003; Hindmarsh and Pilnick, 2002). Looking at what people say and do, millisecond by millisecond, they show that seemingly simple interactions such as the passing of an instrument actually require significant fine-tuning and careful monitoring of the body movements of colleagues. The social semiotic take we propose in this chapter adopts a similar analytical approach, taking seriously the details of different forms of communication, but its theoretical framing is different. Connected with critical discourse analysis and educational studies (Kress and van Leeuwen, 2001), our theory highlights the power relations that shape people's engagement with the world.

The chapter is organised as follows: in the next section, we outline our social semiotic theory of communication and learning; in the following two sections, we expand on some of the key concepts, using examples from clinical and non-clinical sites of learning; we conclude with discussing the implications of our take for learning and assessment in and through clinical practice.

Meaning making, multimodality and power in sites of learning

In all communication, in all domains of the contemporary social world, meanings are made in ensembles consisting of different *modes*: with gestures and speech, with objects, writing, images, gaze, posture and actions all contributing meaning; always with several of these in complex conjunctions. Each of these *modes* offers specific *affordances* – that is, potentials for communication. As a simple example, consider Figure 7.1.

This figure is an excerpt from a surgical textbook discussing how to remove a stone that has been retained in the bile duct following gall bladder removal. Here, *writing* provides a description (a 'recipe') of how to remove a retained stone in the bile duct. For instance, it is explained that 'a wire basket can be passed along the catheter to catch and withdraw the retained calculus'. *Image* provides details that would be difficult or impossible to describe using words. One image is an X-ray depicting a retained stone in the bile duct of a patient. Another image is a drawing depicting how the catheter is spatially arranged in relation to the liver, the intestine, and so on. Without the use of either the one or the other, the information provided by the written account alone would be severely limited, relative to the information needed. That is one of our key premises: that clinicians always draw on a multiplicity of modes to make meaning, whether they write or read a surgical textbook, present a case to a colleague, clerk a patient or operate on a patient.

Social semiotic theory (Kress, 2010; Hodge and Kress, 1988) focuses on *meaning making*, in all modes. The theory brings all socially organised resources that people use to make meaning into one analytical domain. These resources include *modes* such as image, writing, gesture, gaze, speech and posture, and *media* such as screens (of which there are many in clinical settings), forms of various kinds, notes and notebooks. The agency of meaning *makers* in meaning *making* is central. That forces us to think of clinicians as actors in a social world; they make meaning in relation to others, to serve their *interest*, using the resources for making meaning that are available in a particular culture (e.g. a medical culture), on a particular occasion, in a particular site and situation. For instance, in the anaesthetic room, anaesthetists may use *speech* to talk to the patient, for instance

Work-based Learning in Clinical Settings

EBM 18.7 ANTIBIOTIC PROPHYLAXIS IN LAPAROSCOPIC CHOLECYSTECTOMY

'Routine prophylactic administration of antibiotics is unnecessary in patients at low risk of wound or post-operative infection.'
Al-Ghnaniem R, et al. Br J Surg 2003; 90(3):365–366.

hypovolaemic shock. Blood may issue from the drain, if one is present, and re-exploration is mandatory.

18 Infective complications

Wound infection from organisms present in the bile (notably *E. coli, Klebsiella aerogenes* and *Strep. faecalis*) can be reduced following cholecystectomy by the intravenous administration of a cephalosporin at the time of induction of anaesthesia, although the routine use of this group of drugs at laparoscopic cholecystectomy has recently been questioned (EBM 18.7). A longer course of antibiotics may be prescribed when operating on patients with obstructive jaundice, cholangitis, or complications such as acute cholecystitis or empyema when significant bile contamination of the peritoneal cavity has occurred. Collections of bile and/or blood readily become infected after cholecystectomy. Formal drainage may be needed if this progresses to the formation of a subhepatic or subphrenic abscess.

Bile leakage

This may be due to a ligature or clip slipping off the cystic duct, the accidental division of an unrecognized accessory duct, damage to the common bile duct, or retention of a duct stone after exploration. Bile leakage may be evidenced by the development of abnormal LFTs and localized or generalized abdominal pain. It may be contained if a drain is in place. In the absence of biliary peritonitis, a persistent leak requires investigation by means of endoscopic cholangiography. Surgery may be needed if biliary peritonitis develops.

Retained stones

Following bile duct exploration, the post-operative T-tube cholangiogram (see above) may reveal a retained stone in the bile duct. Small stones can sometimes be flushed into the duodenum by irrigating the T-tube with saline, and their passage may be facilitated if glucagon is given to relax the sphincter of Oddi. If the duct cannot be cleared by irrigation, delayed extraction of the stones may be undertaken under radiological control. The patient is discharged with the T-tube in place. This is removed 4–6 weeks later and a steerable catheter passed along its track into the bile duct. A wire (Dormia) basket can be passed along the catheter to catch and withdraw the retained calculus (Fig. 18.23).

In some patients, unsuspected stones may be left in the bile duct at cholecystectomy. Such stones usually give rise to complications such as jaundice, cholangitis and pancreatitis in the months and years following cholecystectomy. ERCP can be used to confirm the presence of such retained stones (Fig. 18.24) and endoscopic papillotomy is performed to recover them (Fig. 18.25). In this technique,

264

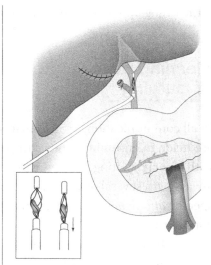

Fig. 18.23 Removal of a retained common bile duct stone.

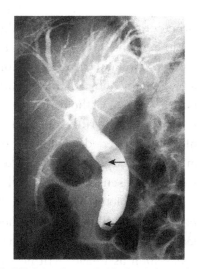

Fig. 18.24 Endoscopic retrograde cholangiography demonstrating multiple stones (arrows) within the biliary tree.
These calculi were removed from the dilated bile duct by balloon extraction following sphincterotomy.

FIGURE 7.1 Excerpt from a surgical textbook (Garden O.J., Bradbury, A. W., Forsythe, J. L. R., *et al.* (2007) *Principles and Practices of Surgery*. 5th edn. Philadelphia, Elsevier, p.264. © 2007 Elsevier; reproduced with permission of Elsevier)

to reassure the patient and explain what they do. As they are talking to the patient they can *gaze* at the operating department practitioner to communicate a request for passing an instrument. As soon as the patient is asleep, speech becomes available again for articulating such requests (see Hindmarsh and Pilnick, 2002).

In research in secondary schools some of us looked at how a 'curriculum', say English or science, is produced within and across modes and media in a class-room: as the teacher's speech, gesture or enactment, as worksheets, as textbooks, in inscriptions on a board and as three-dimensional models (Bezemer and Kress, 2010; Kress *et al.*, 2005; Kress *et al.*, 2001). In that context, we began to see learning as a process of 'principled engagement' with a multimodal environment. A part of learning is understanding the apt resources to bring to bear in a given context to make meanings and then to express meaning: on one occasion a verbal response to the teacher is expected, yet on another, learners are expected to display their engagement through modes other than speech (Bezemer, 2008). This holds true for all meaning makers we observed (in clinical and non-clinical settings), whether as consultant consulting another consultant or as an experienced clinician teaching a relatively inexperienced member of a profession.

In a social semiotic theory, *all* meanings that people make are taken as one kind of evidence of learning. At the same time we acknowledge that not all meaning making 'counts' as learning. We see what counts as learning on a particular occasion – a clinical skills examination, a handover meeting, a ward round – in terms of the *power* of those whose judgement enters at a particular point to decide what shall publicly count as learning, and how it shall be measured. This take is by no means a mainstream view of learning: it is not usual to foreground the power relations that shape learning and ascribe agency to students as well as to teachers in making selections of the 'stuff' to engage with. Present methods of assessment stand as guardians against such a view. In the dominant 'clinical' model of communication, the clinician in power (e.g. the consultant) is seen as the active cause of communication. It is the responsibility of the dominated (the trainee, the patient) to ensure that the 'message' to be 'decoded' is identical with that of the message that was 'encoded' (for detailed observations of how clinicians construct this model in everyday clinical practices see Srikant and Roberts, 1999; Drew and Heritage, 1992). The power of the teacher was/is not in question. By contrast, from our perspective, the responsibility for making meaning of what the 'teacher' says and does lies with the learner; the authority of the teacher is not diminished but it is differently directed and focused.

Communication and learning are always tied to a place. Before clinical trainees start 'doing' clinical work, they will have spent time in classrooms, where teachers give lectures; in 'skills labs', where teachers give demonstrations; and, increasingly, in simulation suites, where they do clinical work without any risk for patients (Bezemer, 2012). And then, of course, there are many different clinical sites: the clinic, the ward, the operating theatre, the trauma bay and so forth. In other words, clinicians 'learn' in many different 'sites'. We take *sites of learning* to be a description from a social perspective of a site, material/physical, formal or informal, immaterial and 'virtual', in which learning 'happens', 'takes place'. In considering sites of learning, our focus is on the *social* organisation of a site – who are the participants, what are their relations, what power is at issue, what social purposes have been assigned to the site, in what ways are they exercised? In that sense, the operating theatre is a site of learning in that it is socially designated for specific social purposes, for a specific group.

Here we want to compare the operating theatre with the home as a 'site of learning', of a father with his 3-year-old child. While these two sites are quite different institutionally and materially, they both show how engagement with the world – which in our theory prompts learning – is socially organised and rendered visible through meanings made by those who inhabit that site. Drawings made by a child and a surgeon, respectively, provide the context for our discussion of the notions of *interest* and *engagement*. The operating theatre, and the body movements and use of speech by a registrar and a medical student, provide the context for our discussion of *design* and *mimesis*. These concepts are applicable to both sites.

Interest and engagement

A 3-year-old, sitting on his father's lap, draws a series of circles, seven to be exact (*see* Figure 7.2). At the end he says: 'this is a car'.

Whether from the perspective of learning or of meaning making, the question arises as to how this is or could be 'a car'. While drawing, he had said 'here's a wheel, here's another wheel, that's a funny wheel.... This is a car'. In other words, for him the criterial feature of a car was its 'wheelness', that it had (many) wheels. Wheels were represented by circles, and 'car' was represented by the arrangement of seven circles. To represent wheels by circles rests on the process of analogy: wheels are like circles. The result of the analogy is a metaphor; similarly, with the representation of car, 'a car is like many wheels'. The meaning made here is a succession of two metaphors: wheels are like circles; and many circles are like a car.

We might ask further why, for this child, wheels could be the criterial feature

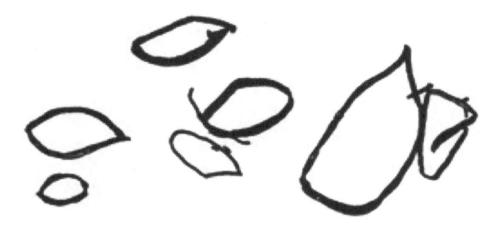

FIGURE 7.2 Drawing by a 3-year-old child

for 'car'. If we imagine the eye level of a 3-year-old looking at the family car (in this case a 1982 Volkswagen Golf, with its prominently visible wheels, especially at that height) we might conclude that this meaning maker's position in the world, literally, physically, but also psychically, affectively, might well lead him to see cars in that way. His drawing, therefore, represents his 'position', his 'interest', arising out of his physical, affective, cultural and social position in the world at that moment, vis-à-vis the object to be represented. From the perspective of learning, we can say that his interest shapes his attention to a part of the world and, in this, acts as a principle for selection (Kress, 1997).

That applies to clinicians as much as to any other social actor. We could have analysed Figure 7.3, a drawing made by a surgical registrar while discussing with a fellow registrar the procedure they are about to carry out. The point we want to make remains the same: it is the *interest* of the meaning maker which determines what is taken as criterial about an entity at the moment of its representation. The surgeon's drawing represents a surgical eye, a 'professional vision' (Goodwin, 1994) of the world; the child's drawing is suggestive of a view of the world that is differently shaped, socially and culturally. What the meaning maker takes as criterial determines what he or she will represent about that entity. Only what is criterial is represented; other features are left out or backgrounded. Hence representation is always partial. That is the case with the 'car' as much as with the representation of the lungs in the top right corner of the surgeon's drawing. The drawings are the result of their work in their *engagement* with their world, embodying their interests.

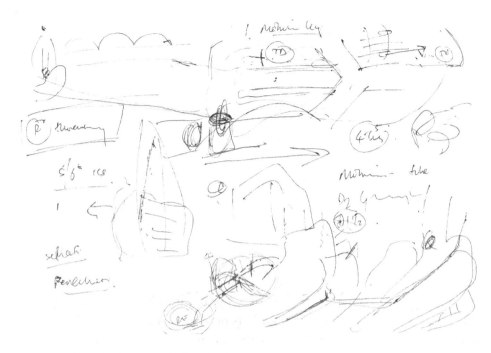

FIGURE 7.3 Drawing by a surgical registrar

Taking the drawings as signs of learning, we suggest that as a result of the process of engagement the child and the surgeon have made new 'concepts', and integrated these into their conceptual resources. Their entire set of resources is transformed in that process, and learning has taken place. They have achieved an augmentation of capacities for representation through making new meanings. Every drawing, indeed any representational form, is new, an innovation, and their making is creative. That (serial) process of *transformative engagement*, integration and transformation, together with its resultant state, constitutes learning. Whether in meaning making or in learning, interest is decisive. It forms the basis: of the choice of what is taken as criterial (in Figure 7.2, the wheels of a car; in Figure 7.3, the carina – that is, the point where the trachea branches out); of the apt means for representation (e.g. a drawing instead of speech); and for transforming that with which the learner has engaged. In learning, the interest of the learner shapes attention to that which is to be learnt, leading to selection from the world, and determines the focus on what is to be engaged with in learning.

Design and mimesis

We now shift to the operating theatre to look at learning involving a different set of modes – speech, body postures, touch and so forth – and a different set of social roles –'lead surgeon' and 'assistant'. Our interest is in how the participants in this site jointly *design* a learning environment using all those modes, and in how learning becomes visible in this environment as a *mimetic* process – that is, as 'creative imitation'.

We focus on a surgical case (para-umbilical hernia repair/excision of lipoma) involving a specialist registrar and a medical student. In our research site, it is not unusual for a registrar to do this procedure independently without the consultant being present, but it is slightly unusual for the registrar to be assisted by a medical student: this would normally be done by a junior postgraduate trainee (e.g. a Foundation Year 2 doctor), possibly with a medical student as a second assistant. However, on the day of this operation, none of the junior postgraduate trainees were available. The registrar stands on the right side of the table, the medical student on the left side, and closer to the leg end of the patient and in front of the instrument trolley stands the scrub nurse; the anaesthetist is seated behind the drape, near the patient's head (*see* Figure 7.4).

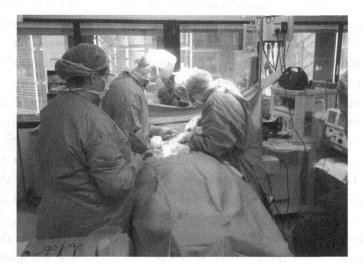

FIGURE 7.4 At the operating table

When the registrar has painted the patient's abdomen with antiseptic, she tells the medical student where to stand and how to jointly unfold the blue drape and place it around the patient's abdomen. She explains how to stick his side of the drape on to the skin, while she positions the drapes. The lump that they will operate on is not visible while the patient is in this flat position. Someone adjusts the operating light, focusing the light on the patient's navel. The nurse hands over the diathermy, an instrument for cutting and coagulating blood to enable dissection. The registrar asks the scrub nurse for a couple of dry swabs while the medical student adjusts his gloves. They then both rest their hands on the patient.

The scrub nurse then provides the requested swabs. With her right hand she picks up a swab from her left hand and places it on the registrar's side of the patient's abdomen. She then drops the swab that remained in her left hand on the medical student's side. The registrar picks up the swab with her right hand and starts dipping it gently onto and just above the area where the lump must be, just below the navel. The medical student picks up the swab closest to him, a split second after the registrar has picked up hers. When the registrar has dipped four times the medical student also has a turn, dipping his swab on to the area just below the navel. However, when his swab comes closer to the skin, the registrar's hand and swab are still there, so they collide. The medical student then withdraws his hand, and the registrar performs one more quick 'dip' before also withdrawing her hand.

The registrar then points with her left hand to where the (invisible) lump that they will operate on is located and asks if he wants to have 'a feel of that'. The medical student replies 'yeah', dipping at three different points around the focal area with the swab in his left hand. He then 'feels' with his right hand. He holds his hand flat, putting gentle pressure on various points with the tip of his fingers, covering an area of about 3 inches below the navel. The registrar then joins him in 'feeling', using her left hand; yet she 'feels' differently. Her hand is slightly tilted, she creates more pressure with the tip of her fingers and the pressure is focused on one point immediately below the navel. This is then followed by a grasping gesture involving her middle finger and her thumb, which lasts for a couple of seconds. Her hand movements suggest that she feels the lump that she is about to operate on, while the medical student's hand movements suggest uncertainty as to what and where to feel.

While the registrar is performing the grasping gesture, she tells the medical student more about the patient: 'When he's awake he has got a small cough impulse and he's a bit tender. But he's had an ultrasound scan which suggests that it's a lipoma. Clinically I think you'd have to say that it's more likely that it's a hernia.' So while she may be feeling the lump, she does not know at this point whether it is a lipoma or a hernia. A lipoma is a fatty lump in the outer layers of the abdominal wall, whereas a hernia is a protrusion of fat or even organs such as small bowel through a defect in the abdominal wall. The registrar refers to her preoperative examination of the patient, suggesting that the lump appears to reduce when relaxed, contradicting the ultrasound scan, which does not show any defects in the abdominal wall. This uncertainty is marked on all written documents circulating in the operating theatre, from checklist to whiteboard, where the name of the procedure is described as 'Abdo wall + Lipoma *or* hernia' [our emphasis].

So while the lump is not nearly as palpable for the medical student as it is for the registrar, they are both faced with uncertainty. In this example, the uncertainty of the medical student is caused by his limited clinical experience, while the uncertainty of the registrar is caused by limitations on diagnostic techniques currently available in medicine. Thus the medical student's hand movements not only 'give off' a sense of uncertainty but also place him in the position of a 'student' who demonstrates that he does not 'know' something. The registrar's spoken comments expressing diagnostic uncertainty do not have the same effect, since at this point in the operation, before the lump has been rendered visible through dissection, no surgeon could have produced a 'legitimate' diagnosis.

Our social semiotic perspective recognises these differences between the medical student and the registrar. In our terminology, they have different access to the socially and culturally shaped resources that count as legitimate in biomedicine. However, we would be reluctant to treat the medical student as the only 'learner' in this example. The medical student may have been the only one to *demonstrate* 'what he still needs to learn' (i.e. which of the resources he has yet got to appropriate), but we *assume* that both the medical student's and the registrar's understandings of the world have changed as a result of the actions and interactions they just engaged in. Those changes go beyond the 'clinical' experience; they affect understandings of not only patients and procedures but also of the people they work with. For instance, what meaning did the registrar attach to the hand movements of the medical student? And how does that meaning shape the learning environment?

Answers to such questions may not always be readily available. Sometimes one cannot identify *signs of learning*, or one cannot be certain what change is demonstrated in communication. However, that does not mean the changes have not taken place, or that such questions do not need to be asked. Let's look at what happens after the registrar's diagnostic account. The registrar now opens the skin and provides a spoken commentary at the same time, explaining how to start an incision, where to put swabs, which setting on the diathermy device to use for which parts of the incision, and so forth. Thus she uses speech to draw the attention of the medical student to some of the actions she performs, while leaving out others. This selection is shaped by and suggestive of the registrar's interest and her understanding of the medical student. If his touching had appeared more like her own, the registrar would probably have drawn his attention to something that she believed was more 'apt' for a learner whose clinical experience was closer to hers. In that, she demonstrates her 'learning' about this student.

Clinicians often think of the spoken commentary provided by the registrar as 'teaching'. Indeed, it is a deliberate attempt by the registrar to guide the medical student's engagement with the world, suggesting what to attend to and in what order. His ignoring of this guidance would again shape the registrar's understanding of the medical student, and probably not in a constructive way. Thus these teaching episodes highlight the agency of the 'teacher' – in this case, the registrar – and they highlight the episodes that involve speech. Most of the clinicians who we talked to at our research site see this as evidence of the fact that teaching is provided mainly or even exclusively through speech. This belief often goes hand in hand with the notions of 'implicitness' and 'explicitness', whereby 'teaching' is seen as 'making explicit' (through speech) that which is implicit in the work of those who are already full members of the profession.

Instead our notion of *design* acknowledges that learning environments are created using not only speech but also gesture, gaze, body posture and so forth. We have already seen examples of that. The registrar points at the area just below the navel before inviting the medical student to 'have a feel'. This pointing is not only a precursor of the invitation; it also draws the student's attention to the area he ought to feel. We have observed many such examples, including ones where speech was not involved at all. In those cases, people would, for example, cut a suture or dissect a piece of tissue held by others in response to pointing gestures (see Bezemer *et al.*, 2011b, for a detailed description of these examples). Following our concept of 'affordance', we see all of these embodied actions, not only speech, as 'explications'. The different forms of representation and communication have distinctive potentials and constraints, and so clinicians use them to make different things explicit, rather than 'translating' into speech what is already 'implicitly there' in other modes. The pointing gesture of the registrar, for instance, is a precise explication of an area that is left unspecified in the co-occurring question, 'do you wanna have a feel?' At the same time, the pointing gesture alone does not constitute a complete invitation to the medical student to 'have a feel'.

Our example not only shows *what* the medical student is learning (namely, how to feel); it also shows *how* he learns. We have already seen this in our example, when the registrar and the medical student were both dipping the patient's skin dry. When she rests her hands on the patient while asking for a couple of swabs from the scrub nurse, he too rests his hands on the patient. When she picks up a swab, he does too. When she starts dipping, he does too. This demonstrates the *mimetic* character of learning. In the words of Christoph Wulf (Wulf *et al.*, 2010), mimesis is 'creative imitation':

> Mimetic learning is productive; it is related to the body, and it establishes a connection between the individual and the world as well as other persons; it creates practical knowledge, which is what makes it constitutive of social, artistic, and practical action. (p.xv)

Mimesis takes us away from the notion of teaching and the agency it places on the side of the teacher. It highlights the agency of learners in terms of what they choose to engage with, especially if there are no 'teachers' around to guide them through design. We can illustrate this with an example from the same operation. Previously we discussed the registrar making a skin incision and giving a spoken commentary. When the incision is complete, a new stage in the operation begins, requiring different manual actions, a different set of instruments, and, consequently, a new division of labour. Retractors now need to be placed and held in position so that registrar and medical student can dissect around the lump. The first time round, the registrar places the retractors and then hands them over to the medical student (without actually *saying* anything). If she needs the medical student to provide a slightly different kind of traction she holds on to his hand and adjusts its position (again without saying anything).

There are two points here: on the one hand, the 'teaching' surgeon teaches by action where that is the better suited mode; on the other hand, this is a typical social organisation of surgical work – a senior surgeon does the 'invasive' work, while her or his assistants hold things up, pull things aside, and so forth. What is less typical, but what happened in our example, is that from instance to instance increasingly, the medical student places and replaces the retractors himself, mimicking what he saw the registrar doing moments earlier. The registrar soon acknowledges this new role by *asking* him to place the retractors instead of placing them herself or repositioning his hand. For instance, she points at the retractor held in his right hand and asks him to 'slide that in laterally'. This is how power relations are negotiated, shifting the initial enactment of 'teacher' and 'learning assistant' to 'lead surgeon' and 'assistant' and redistributing the agency of the two actors involved in this clinical work.

Implications for learning and assessment
••

We have reviewed two sites of learning in some detail. The first was a home, and the social roles involved in the interaction between the inhabitants of that site were a father and his son. The focus of our analysis was on a drawing made by the son. The drawing showed to what in the world the son's attention was drawn, relatively independent of the interests of the father. The second was an operating theatre, and some of the roles enacted here were a registrar and a medical student. Our analytical focus was on the body positioning and movement, in particular of the hands, and the speech used by them. The communication between them showed what it was in the world to which the attention of the registrar and the medical student was drawn, and how their orientations were mutually shaping.

It is at this point where a social semiotic multimodal theory widens our perspective on learning and resets the frame for what we should attend to. Meaning making happens everywhere and all the time, not only when 'taught', 'instructed', or otherwise 'organised', 'set up', 'designed' for learning, whether in a seminar room or when 'at work'. Meanings are made in any mode, not just speech, and all meaning making constitutes a sign of learning. That sheds a different light on notions of 'explicitness' and 'implicitness'. From a social semiotic perspective, these notions are social and cultural categories, not intrinsic properties of forms of representation. In 'Western' societies, so-called, these notions have had far-reaching effects on mainstream and dominant conceptions of teaching, learning and assessment. What could be spoken, written, represented in numerical form or as formulae has been treated as explicit knowledge. Much other 'knowing' – being implicit – was thought to be beyond overt teaching or deliberate learning. That had led to a 'naturalising' of the practices at work in the social construction of the profession: certain definitional things, it was assumed, could not be taught, and that in turn led to the folksy common sense idea that, say, a '"real" journalist, writer, surgeon is born not made'.

A multimodal social semiotic approach to knowing opens the door to making 'unspoken knowing' audible and visible, to understanding *embodied* learning and teaching. With that, the frame around what 'can' and what 'cannot' be taught and how, in any case 'things might be learned' has been expanded enormously. Speech as much as writing assumes a new place in the semiotic landscape: expressing certain things exceedingly well, but coming to the limits of their capacity when pushed to writing out how to intubate a patient. Here the physical guiding of the arms and hands of the learner by the experienced anaesthetist proves to be by far the superior route to knowing in embodied teaching and learning. *Multimodality* provides descriptions and accounts of all these forms of meaning and knowing. *Social semiotics* focuses on and highlights the agency of the individual, expressed through the interest of the meaning maker in which his or her engagement with the world is paramount. This opens up both a vast challenge for notions and practices of assessment and evaluation and the need for a full awareness of the *means of recognition* of learning. If learning is not recognised, it cannot be evaluated.

Above all, a multimodal social semiotic approach offers the possibility of moving on from distinctions such as 'implicit' or 'tacit' and 'explicit' learning, and 'hidden' and 'explicit' curricula. When first used, these distinctions served to highlight the working of power in education. Over time, we have begun to take these distinctions for granted, losing sight of fundamental questions such as, What actually *is* implicit learning? *Who* hides which curriculum? These are questions of politics and power that translate into ontologies and epistemologies. If education, whether in schools or workplaces, is to produce conformity and adherence to convention, then notions of correctness and of error will prevail. If the aim is to understand the transformative engagement of learners, then other notions will need to prevail, predominantly those of interest and meaning making. That would lead to entirely different forms and conceptions of assessment than those of conformity to power in its manifold forms. That is the case whatever the environments of learning might be.

Environments of clinical learning are in the process of undergoing changes of the most profound kind, largely externally produced. Conceptions of learning, teaching and assessment will need to become adequate for the demands posed by current and future environments of learning. Making the currently inaudible audible, the invisible visible and the implicit open to recognition is crucial in that process.

Acknowledgements

We are grateful to all National Health Service staff who welcomed us in their operating theatres. We would also like to thank the funders of our project, 'Mapping Educational Activity in the Operating Theatre'. They are the Royal College of Surgeons of England, which funded a research fellowship (2009–10), and the London Deanery, which granted an award under the Simulation and Technology-Enhanced Learning Initiative (2009–12).

References

Bezemer, J. (2008) Displaying orientation in the classroom: students' multimodal responses to teacher instructions. *Linguistics and Education*, 19(2), 166–78.

Bezemer, J. (2012) Learning, design and performance: towards a semiotic-ethnographic account of surgical simulation. In: N. Pachler and M. Böck (eds) *Multimodality and Social Semiotics: communication, meaning-making and learning in the work of Gunther Kress*. New York, NY, Routledge.

Bezemer, J. and Kress, G. (2010) Changing text: a social semiotic analysis of textbooks. *Designs for Learning*, 3(1–2), 10–29.

Bezemer, J., Cope, A., Kress, G., *et al.* (2011a) 'Do you have another Johan?' Negotiating meaning in the operating theatre. *Applied Linguistics Review*, 2, 313–34.

Bezemer, J., Murtagh, G., Cope, A., *et al.* (2011b) 'Scissors, please': the practical accomplishment of surgical work in the operating theatre. *Symbolic Interaction*, 34(3), 398–414.

Drew, P. and Heritage, J. (1992) *Talk at Work: interaction in institutional settings*. Cambridge, Cambridge University Press.

Goodwin, C. (1994) Professional vision. *American Anthropologist*, 96(3), 606–33.

Heath, C., Hindmarsh, J. and Luff, P. (2010) *Video in Qualitative Research: analysing social interaction in everyday life*. London, Sage.

Hindmarsh, J. and Pilnick, A. (2002) The tacit order of teamwork: collaboration and embodied conduct in anaesthesia. *Sociological Quarterly*, 43(2), 139–64.

Hodge, B. and Kress, G. (1988) *Social Semiotics*. Cambridge, Polity.

Iedema, R., Long, D., Forsyth, R., *et al.* (2006) Visibilising clinical work: video ethnography in the contemporary hospital. *Health Sociology Review*, 15(2), 156–68.

Kissmann, U. (ed) (2009) *Video Interaction Analysis: methods and methodology*. Frankfurt, Peter Lang.

Koschmann, T., LeBaron, C., Goodwin, C., *et al.* (2011) 'Can you see the cystic artery yet?' A simple matter of trust. *Journal of Pragmatics*, 43(2), 521–41.

Kress, G. (1997) *Before Writing: rethinking the paths to literacy*. London, Routledge.

Kress, G. (2010) *Multimodality: a social semiotic approach to contemporary communication*. London, Routledge.

Kress, G. and van Leeuwen, T. (2001) *Multimodal Discourse: the modes and media of contemporary communication*. London, Routledge.

Kress, G., Charalampos, T., Jewitt, C., *et al.* (2001) *Multimodal Teaching and Learning: the rhetorics of the science classroom*. London, Continuum.

Kress, G., Jewitt, C., Bourne, J., *et al.* (2005) *English in Urban Classrooms: a multimodal perspective on teaching and learning*. London, Routledge Farmer.

Lave, J. and Wenger, E. (1991) *Situated Learning: legitimate peripheral participation*. Cambridge, Cambridge University Press.

Lingard, L., Espin, S., Whyte, S., *et al.* (2004) Communication failures in the operating room: an observational classification of recurrent types and effects. *Quality and Safety in Health Care*, 13(5), 330–4.

Mondada, L. (2003) Working with video: how surgeons produce video records of their actions. *Visual Studies*, 18(1), 58–73.

Säljö, R. (2009) *The Conceptualization of Learning in Learning Research: from experimental introspectionism and conditioned reflexes to meaning-making and performativity in situated practices*. Unpublished paper, University of Gothenburg.

Srikant, S. and Roberts, C. (1999) *Talk, Work and Institutional Order: discourse in medical, mediation and management settings*. Berlin, Mouton de Gruyter.

Svensson, M.S., Heath, C. and Luff. P. (2007) Instrumental action: the timely exchange of implements during surgical operations. In: L. Bannon, I. Wagner, C. Gutwin, *et al.* (eds) *Proceedings of the 10th European Conference on Computer-Supported Cooperative Work*. Limerick, Springer, pp.41–60.

Wulf, C., Aithans, B. and Audehm, K. (2010) *Ritual and Identity: the staging and performing of rituals in the lives of young people*. London, Tufnell.

8

Establishing patient safety nets

How actor-network-theory can inform clinical education research

Alan Bleakley

Prologue

Imagine: you are sitting in the bath reading this chapter. Normally, you look forward to this relaxing moment, this mini-holiday, an opportunity for time out in a hectic day when you can also fully concentrate without distraction. However, it is late, you are overtired, the bath is neither hot nor full enough, you cannot settle into a comfortable position to read, and you are now irritated that you have not got the hang of the paragraph you have just read. Nevertheless, from the late evening's ruins, a nascent idea dawns, and you want to get it down before it evaporates – but you do not have a notebook and pen handy! You go back to the paragraph and read it again, but find yourself drifting and nodding with tiredness so that you nearly let the book fall out of your hands. You come back to reality with a jolt, the edge of your expensive and once-pristine book now stained with bathwater. The book suddenly feels very heavy and awkward to hold.

Your idea, in the absence of notebook and pen, has already dissolved, along with your patience, and now your book is close to following the same course, as your concentration is shot. This lost learning scenario is ripe for analysis through actor-network-theory. There was no Archimedes-style 'Eureka!' moment. Rather, the glimmer of an idea dissolved where a network failed to form. The initiation of a network offers a potential transformation, but you are dead in the water. Your body was tired and your concentration poor and this was aggravated by having to hold up what felt like an increasingly heavy book. There was no paper or pen at hand.

What is the point of this depressing little story? First, context matters where learning is concerned. Second, context centrally involves objects – artefacts such as the contours of your bath, the temperature of the bathwater and the shape and weight of the book you are reading. These are, in actor-network-theory, all significant 'actors' in the drama of learning. I am introducing them early in this chapter so that their significance will not be forgotten. On another day, the context may not have bitten back, but rather acted to promote learning, as a network was formed in a stream of connections between hot bathwater, engaging book, relaxed body and buzzing brain.

Part I: the architecture of actor-network-theory

Introduction

Actor-network-theory (hereafter 'ANT') resists reduction to a concise description. Bruno Latour's (2007) so-called 'Introduction' to ANT is a closely argued text of 300 pages. However, Akrich *et al.* (2002, p.205) offer a concise account of ANT as a research method, where they say that 'Innovation is the art of interesting an increasing number of allies who will make you stronger and stronger'. Where ANT-inspired clinical education research makes claims for promoting innovation, knowledge production and transformation of practices, this can be summarised as the formation, and subsequent widening and strengthening, of a learning network. What, however, is a 'network'? And who or what are the 'allies' that must be increased or enrolled to make a network stronger? We have already seen that such 'allies' can include the temperature of your bathwater.

ANT offers an apology

ANT has acquired a potentially unhelpful mystique as a left-field approach, offering 'a body of unsettling and rather audacious work' that operates 'around the edges of educational research' and sets out to 'rupture central assumptions' within educational theory (Fenwick and Edwards, 2010, p.viii). The rhetoric is clear and the supporting metaphors powerful: 'unsettling' and 'audacious', 'edges' and 'ruptures'. We expect to find ourselves at our limits, the ground taken from under our feet.

We would feel that we were on reasonably safe ground if someone explained that ANT involved 'actors', 'networks' and 'theory', and, as the hyphens suggest, that these are linked in some way. It was therefore disconcerting when Latour (1999) – the single most influential voice in ANT – famously announced that there are four things wrong with ANT – 'actor', 'network', 'theory' and the hyphen! (Originally Latour only used the first hyphen in the term.) Latour's tongue was not in his cheek – rather, he feared that ANT would be reduced to a formulaic approach and misinterpreted in the process, the acronym coming to act as an aphorism or an old saw – a pithy statement supposedly embodying wisdom, but paradoxically disembowelling wisdom.

In a later overview of ANT, however, Latour (2007) offers an apology for his earlier rather grumpy decision, recognising that where use of the acronym is widespread, he may as well turn it into a virtue. 'ANT', suggests Latour (2007, p.9), is 'so awkward, so confusing, so meaningless that it deserves to be kept', on the basis that it is a good descriptor for a 'myopic, workaholic, trail-sniffing, and collective traveler'. For good measure, Latour added another hyphen (from the convention of 'actor-network theory' to 'actor-network-theory') to further emphasise linkage between the components. In this chapter, I follow Latour's sentiment and prefer to keep my own nose close to the ground, mainly for the rich research detail that this posture affords. I also retain Latour's usage of the double hyphen, to stress that actor-network-theory is a linked whole, a world view and way of being, exceeding the limitations of an applied technique. Later in the chapter, however, I will point out some key objections to ANT, signifying limitations to its use within clinical education and its research arm.

The second hyphen in actor-network-theory also serves to repair the historical separation of theory and practice. ANT can be taken as an example of what Schatzki *et al.* (2001) describe as 'the practice turn in contemporary theory', where theory is *performed*. Mind and knowledge are constituted and social life is organised and transformed through action and interaction, or activity. ANT is not an analytical apparatus but 'more like a sensibility, an interruption or intervention, a way to sense and draw nearer to a phenomenon' (Fenwick and Edwards, 2010, p.ix). Medicine is often characterised as an Aristotelian *phronesis* – a 'practical wisdom' (Bleakley *et al.*, 2011) – and medical education and its research arm are consequently infected with such pragmatism. With its emphasis upon educating sensibility rather than analytical reasoning, ANT would seem to afford a ready-made pragmatic research approach for medical education, and it is puzzling that its uptake has not been more vigorous within this field of inquiry.

What are actors and networks and how do they link?

In ANT, 'actor' refers to any phenomenon – human, material object (artefact) or concept (the imaginary, ideas). Phenomena in self-presentation are irreducible to any other expression – such as higher order categories – so ANT researchers resist drawing, first, on grand theoretical frames (such as Marxism or psychoanalysis) that shape or prejudge data collection; and, second, on the use of themes in data analysis, typically employed to order otherwise disorderly data. Fenwick and Edwards (2010, p.146) suggest that 'What ANT brings to its ethnographic methodological approaches is a sensibility for mess and it attempts to suspend a priori assumptions'. The ground rule is to stick with (and to) the mess in closely following the actors.

Because 'actor' is associated with persons in the English language, ANT also uses 'actant'. Throughout this chapter, I will refer to actors. Actors interact in meaningful and non-meaningful ways. For ANT, a meaningful interaction is where one actor has an effect upon another (e.g. a mobile phone ringtone captures the attention of somebody who is daydreaming) to realise a *transformation*, a change of state, an innovation or a production of knowledge. This linkage is dynamic, moving through time. ANT calls this a 'translation', because the actors involved are now no longer the same as before.

The actors are mediators of this process of translation, or are affected by the movement of translation. For example, the person answers the mobile phone to discover that her best friend has just died in a car accident, at which point a potential, and emotionally painful, network is initiated. If the actors are linked but no translation occurs, then a network fails to form. In the example given, the person may have missed the call. Where actors interact without transformation (such as automatically deleting spam mail), they act as 'intermediaries' rather than 'mediators'. Educational activity for ANT is a mediated network effect – a series of mutual translations between actors leading to transformation such as adoption of a new work practice. ANT is a way of accounting for how persons, material objects and ideas become linked as fluid networks through tracing effects generated by the 'work' that is the assembling and strengthening of the network. ANT's concerns are inevitably 'work based'.

Symmetry among humans, material objects and immaterial languages

ANT's key philosophical contribution is the radical notion of *generalised symmetry* – where all phenomena, whether human, material or semiotic, are afforded equal ontological status within a network effect (Harman, 2009). This notion separates ANT from other approaches to clinical education, where both objects and concepts are often given secondary ontological status to persons, or only the talk and activities of persons are recorded, as if the world of material objects that these persons interact with is of little consequence. Where the human is figured as having equal ontological status with magnetic resonance imaging scanners, libraries, cutlery and ocean currents, ANT is often referred to as a 'posthuman' outlook (Schatzki *et al.*, 2001).

This radical idea of generalised symmetry has important consequences for clinical education. For example, in studies of practices of 'care', Annemarie Mol (Mol *et al.*, 2010; Mol, 2008) challenges the habitual opposition of 'cold' technologies and 'warm' humans, to demonstrate that health 'care' is usually a product of interaction between the warmth of technologies (e.g. giving oxygen) and the warmth of persons (the nurse adjusting the oxygen mask). To this we can add the potential warmth of the symbol, such as the reassurance signified by the nurse's uniform.

Shifting focus away from just persons (as actors) affords the opportunity to appreciate both the complex and multiple appearances and translations of objects, as they interact with persons through codes and languages, as an ontological effect. The notion of multiple ontologies – states of being – is illustrated by the instability of complex objects of research across contexts. In studying the management of alcoholic liver disease, Law and Singleton (2005) report that keeping this object (the 'illness') to a single meaning is impossible as it comes in and out of focus according to the context in which it appears. Rather than seeing this as a methodological failure, the authors suggest that research methods are ill-equipped to study messy objects. Mol (1999) offers a multiple ontological reading of anaemia, where the condition is 'performed' in at least three different ways: clinically (through medical diagnosis and treatment), pathophysiologically (through laboratory routines) and statistically (through epidemiological analysis).

In a later extensive study, Mol (2002) tracks the diagnosis and treatment of atherosclerosis by a variety of practitioners in a Dutch university hospital. Her ethnography reveals that what is described to patients in information leaflets as 'the gradual obstruction of the arteries' is conceived differently by doctors, vascular surgeons and nurses, and is further modulated by differing professional and lay languages, and through varieties of imaging artefacts such as microscopes, X-rays and ultrasound. By taking, for example, the perspective not only of the human but also of the blood, as this is configured in contexts such as the haematology laboratory, Mol problematises the study of the illness. Here, 'atherosclerosis is enacted as deviance that involves the blood clotting mechanism', and where the patient's blood now flows across a variety of investigative sites, its 'anatomical location is completely lost' (Mol, 2002, p.109).

ANT is drawn to suspect and problematic research contexts, from failures and fault lines to 'black boxes' – habitual or routine activities that disguise complexities such as multiple ontologies. ANT wrestles with the contents of the black box, typically 'tokens' or 'quasi-objects' that are reifications. Examples in clinical education research include terms such as 'teams' (Engeström, 2008) and clinical 'guidelines' (Gabbay and Le May, 2011), used as if they were transparent and had commonly agreed meanings but are actually problematic, concealing more than they reveal.

Without entertaining the radically democratic notion of generalised symmetry, the practices of ANT will never be properly understood. Indeed, as the main philosophical position, generalised symmetry can be taken as the 'theory', conceptual architecture or organising framework, shaping, informing and developing the practices of ANT, bringing actors into significant relationships as network effects. Generalised symmetry can be equated with the hyphens in actor-network-theory, which act not only as links to turn the individual components into a whole but also as mediators or translators (actors form networks and afford theory), and, finally, as levellers, or signifiers of democracy, where actors (persons, artefacts and languages), the networks they form, and the theory they produce to explain and further strengthen such networks, *potentially* have equal power or potency.

What are networks?

As one actor acts upon or mobilises another as a work of translation (so that the actors are both now transformed, as mediators) a network is initiated. Further translations expand the network through alliances. However, 'network' is neither a tangible structure nor a diagrammatic representation. It is a metaphor through which we give meaning to the series of translations that occur as actors work transformatively on other actors.

Networks involve things but are not things themselves, or resist reification. As unpredictable processes, networks cannot be studied like blood samples under the microscope, yet everything realised by the network effect can be treated as concrete and sensible – as things that happen, present themselves to the senses or mind, or can be measured by instrumentation, including floating concepts and intuitive leaps, as well as cold steel and congealing blood. As a dynamic net effect of a series of actor translations and transformations that the researcher attempts to partially retrace, a network is then a net *working* whose echo we closely observe through fieldwork and re-member through research reports.

'Network' as ANT understands it, is unfortunately overshadowed by the black box of the 'Internet', that does not usually act as a dynamic network. When I visit a website for information, buy from an online catalogue or send an email, neither myself nor the website is necessarily transformed in the process. I am usually an intermediary in a predictable consumer exchange and reproduction of knowledge and values, rather than a mediator effecting change, innovation or production of knowledge and values. What has occurred is transaction rather than translation. For ANT, a network goes beyond transaction, as a traceable 'set of relations defined as so many translations' (Latour, 2007, p.129).

Latour (2007) now prefers to call the problematic tracing of the translations across phenomena a *work-net* rather than a network. The emphasis turns from a passive network waiting to be used (a telephone, electricity or sewage system; pipelines; the Internet as a web of computers and exchange sites) to an active web permanently in construction, requiring 'work' both to maintain its momentum (search) and to record its traces (re-search). Latour (2007, p.132) then makes a distinction between the work-net as 'active mediator' and the network as a 'stabilized set of intermediaries'. In ANT research, one must work on and at the fluid net to apprehend the 'trace left behind by some moving agent'. ANT research, as applied to clinical education, is necessarily concerned with 'work'-based learning, where labour can be material (relocating a dislocated shoulder) or immaterial (puzzling out a dislocated sentence uttered by a confused patient).

If a formula for ANT research work were to be proposed, it would be to dramatically increase the relative proportion of mediators to intermediaries, going against the grain of the usual state of affairs where intermediaries will far outweigh mediators. Another way of putting this is that life is mainly a series of *events* (equivalent to 'intermediaries') that fail to promote innovation. Where events turn to *experiences* (equivalent to 'mediators'), something deep happens in the way of learning. Often, a mediator is troublesome or irksome, already getting under the skin, to turn an event into an experience. Here, ANT reformulates Harold Garfinkel's ethnomethodology (1967), which explicitly sets out to problematise the social contexts it researches. Ethnomethodologists deliberately breach social rules and conventions through planned interventions, such as cheating at board games, or acting as a stranger in one's own home, to record reactions.

Rather than intervening in terms of the researcher breaching a convention (which may also have ethical implications), ANT researchers seize upon social phenomena that are already inverted, divisive or calamitous. For example, Latour (1996) studied the conception, but ultimate failure, of a project in Paris for a rapid public transport system – Aramis – showing how a potential network could be initiated but not maintained, so that the project was abandoned as sterile. The frustration of possible translations across actors may cause a potential network to falter. In the Aramis case, this was an economic-technological-political hitch – complicated engineered couplings proved too expensive to produce, and there was a parallel failure of coupling in lack of political support for the project despite a public will.

Feasibility

In such a retracing of the work-net, and having decided that its focus will be inclusive, how does an ANT approach make such a study manageable? Surely, any social phenomenon under investigation is always too complex and its manifestations too numerous to offer any kind of comprehensive account? ANT does not seek a comprehensive account but a close description of a slice of activity, getting so close to the ground that an overview is impossible. ANT research prides itself on its radical localism, suggesting that 'generalisability' in research is a convenient fiction, where all research projects are necessarily local and situated. Will an ANT study then either miss the point completely by its self-inflicted myopia, or will it get lost, indeed suffocate, in excessive detail?

Fortunately, ANT has addressed such questions of scale. To achieve focus, as mentioned earlier, ANT places two primary restrictions upon the study of the initiation, development and future of a work-net/network or a series of interacting networks. First, ANT research focuses upon the work of actors as mediators rather than intermediaries. It is interested in transformations promising innovation, rather than the maintenance of the status quo. Second, ANT chooses to research what is already showing symptoms, signs of wear and tear, instability or a fault line. ANT feeds off controversies, even fiascos. ANT is then selective of the slice of activity for study, but this may be the only explicit marker you will find of its research 'design'.

Where ANT research focuses upon the apparently unremarkable or routine, such as Mol's interest in anaemia, it is because a black box has been opened to expose complexities and contradictions. ANT is sceptical of linear, problem-solving approaches and the hunt for final solutions that together constitute a genre of research typified by the hero's journey – where monsters, riddles and labyrinths are rendered unproblematic and the Grail is revealed or the Minotaur slain.

Part II: let's go to work! Actor-network-theory as a research methodology
••••••••••••••••••••••••••••••••

Introduction

In this section, I describe how an ongoing collaborative inquiry focused upon improving teamwork across operating theatres in one UK teaching hospital has been informed and shaped by an ANT sensibility (Allard *et al.*, 2007; Henderson *et al.*, 2007; Bleakley, 2006a, 2006b; Bleakley *et al.*, 2006; Hobbs, 2005; Hobbs and Bleakley, 2005; Bleakley *et al.*, 2004). The inquiry – the Theatre Team Resource Management (hereafter TTRM) project – was conceived in 2001–02 and initiated in December 2002 to progressively assemble a patient safety work-net/network through strategic alliances focused on a common object: incremental sophistication of communication between team members within the operating theatre (hereafter OT) and across peri-operative environments.

TTRM has been gathered as an open-access website (www.ttrm.co.uk). The website will be updated to include interactive elements, continuing to strengthen the network through a technological ally, and has been adopted by the hospital trust concerned as a platform for developing a rolling in-house staff development programme. This offers an opportunity to develop stronger strategic alliances, particular with trust management, in supporting practice development and innovation. However, strengthening the work-net/network has inevitably invited resistances, threatening ruptures, detailed here along with successful alliances.

Research projects tend to be reported as if they were discrete, ahistorical events. A project of course has a life cycle. There are initial grant applications to be made (including unsuccessful bids, where potential networks remain unrealised), grant obligations to be fulfilled, steering committees to be set up and dissolved, interim and final reports to be submitted, researchers to be appointed to short-term posts, PhD theses to be completed and examined, journal papers, conference presentations and so forth. All projects are necessarily punctuations in a bigger narrative.

Further, as practice changes are adopted and absorbed by the clinical community involved, they become hybrids, locally adapted and mutable. For example, while we modelled, early in the study, an ideal pre-list team-building briefing, at least five local hybrids evolved, including nurses leading the brief in the day case unit and one surgeon developing a 'horizon' brief a week before lists, scanning potential issues. These hybrids have now been eclipsed by the introduction of a mandatory briefing protocol – the World Health Organization's Surgical Safety

Checklist (Gawande, 2009), which itself is destined to be locally adapted and sometimes resisted.

The TTRM project tracks the cumulative impact of a number of collaborative changes in activity on the ethos of the OT as a basis for improving patient safety. The 'interruption' to habitual work practices promises a culture change in communication style, from autocratic and hierarchical patterns to democratic, participatory and dialogical patterns (Bleakley *et al.*, 2011). While ANT's approach is less interventionist and more about interruption, it readily aligns with the values of collaborative inquiry, to research *with* and not *on* practitioners. Practices researched in this context include collaborative briefing and debriefing, before and after a surgical list.

Problematisation

ANT is drawn to conundrums, including practices that are historically crystallised, lacking innovation. Cultural-historical activity theory (CHAT) (*see* Chapter 5, by Clare Morris) is a close companion of ANT. CHAT's major proponent, Yrjö Engeström (1999), describes how in activity research

> [a] new theoretical idea or concept is initially produced in the form of an abstract, simple explanatory relationship, a 'germ cell'. This initial abstraction is step-by-step enriched and transformed into a concrete system of multiple, constantly developing manifestations. In an expansive learning cycle, the initial simple idea is transformed into a complex object, into a new form of practice. At the same time, the cycle produces new theoretical concepts. (p.5)

An example of this process in action can be drawn from the TTRM project. The core research team argued that the assumption among surgical teams that only the lead surgeon could initiate a team briefing should be challenged on the basis that briefing was centrally about establishing team morale, and mutual situational awareness (where each member of the team comes to understand other members' roles in a mini-rehearsal of the day's work ahead). This is Engeström's 'germ cell'. As this abstraction was turned into practice, where, for example, nurses led briefings, this challenged assumptions about autocracy as the default political position for the surgical team, to be replaced by participative democracy. As this was further tested, e.g. with nurses progressively leading briefing as the norm in day case surgery, so objections to such a model from surgeons were challenged and dismissed.

The initial idea is now established through expansion of the learning cycle, as anaesthetists and surgeons begin to see the value of the nurse leading a briefing, where the nurse is already the centre for information exchange and the first stop for patients in the day case unit's extended team. As the practice is developed, so nurses reformulate identities as team leaders, transforming the initial idea into a complex practice that has the immediate effect of collectively raising morale among nurses, but also implies the need for parallel, tailored professional development. Theoretical gain emerges from the process of expansion of the activity of briefing, where surgical teams can now be seen to be experimenting with new forms of work-based democracy, and the identity construction of the nurse is positively and radically reformulated.

The activity cycles of expansive learning in CHAT and the strengthening of networks in ANT act as neither sponges nor cookers – respectively cleaning up and processing raw data. ANT likes its data rare, challenging research studies that draw on a variety of tactics and rhetorical devices to disguise the messy in research that is, after all, a slice of messy life. By 'rare', I mean data that are not overly analysed or processed ('cooked' would be an alternative here, but not in the sense of manipulating data unethically, to purposefully mislead). A model for this kind of research account is Mol's account of the relationships between people living with diabetes and those professionals who care for them (Mol, 2008). Mol derives an argument that critically addresses the logic of 'patient choice' by showing how such logic, in the cases of the diabetics she follows, often frustrates rather than facilitates good care practices. The argument is derived elegantly from the fieldwork – which exposes multiple ontologies – without the mediation of an overwrought epistemology or predisposing framework that may provide a fog to obscure the objects of the research.

Latour (2007, pp.146–7) notes that approaching research analytically is premature: 'we are in the business of descriptions. … we go, we listen, we learn … it's called inquiries. Good inquiries always produce a lot of new descriptions', where 'if your description needs an explanation, it's not a good description'. Conventional research texts often deliberately bracket out context, such as the political, historical and organisational. ANT texts lean towards thick descriptions and baroque detail.

The design of the TTRM project has its origin in an ethical dilemma. While sometimes high risk, surgery has an unacceptably high rate of error; this is grounded not in technical mistakes but in poor communication. An estimated 70% of medical errors result from miscommunications within and between teams and 50% of this is thought to be remediable through improving communication (Pronovost and Vohr, 2010; Kohn *et al.*, 1999). Better clinical teamwork in hospitals correlates with lower morbidity and mortality rates and high levels of work morale (West and Borrill, 2002). Improving communication and teamwork in the OT should ultimately benefit patient safety and challenge work practices that jeopardise patient safety. Engeström (1999) suggests:

> The expansive cycle begins with individual subjects questioning the accepted practice, and it gradually expands into a collective movement or institution. The theory of expansive learning is related to Latour's actor-network theory in that both regard innovations as stepwise construction of new forms of collaborative practice, or technoeconomic networks. (p.5)

In a first round of surveys of 300+ OT staff in 2003 as part of the wider TTRM research that included elements of inquiry other than ANT, we found that perceptions concerning quality of communication differed across professional groups. For example, where 90% of consultant surgeons said that they had good communication with their surgical colleagues, only 50% of consultant anaesthetists, 40% of nurses and 25% of trainee anaesthetists reported that they had good communication with consultant surgeons. When asked how often a pre-list briefing occurs, 10% of surgeons said 'never', 50% 'occasionally' and 40% 'always'. However, when anaesthetists were asked, 70% said 'never', 20% 'occasionally' and 10% 'always'. So what model of 'briefing' did those surgeons hold and whom did they imagine they were briefing? We meticulously followed this fault line.

When we carried out an intensive audit on briefing practices soon after this survey, we found no OT teams which held a properly structured whole-team brief; 'briefing' was often configured as, literally, a brief conversation between the surgeon and anaesthetist, and not a team meeting. Five years after introducing our ANT-inspired 'interruption' with OT allies, an audit showed that 20% of surgical teams were regularly briefing and 15% debriefing, but that 50% of individual practitioners reported having been part of a brief that week, and 30% part of a debrief that week. Given what we know about the pace of practice change in conservative surgical environments, this was relatively good news.

In terms of initiating and strengthening a work-net/network through strategic alliances, we knew how problematic this could be in the face of a surgical culture grounded in hierarchy and meritocracy focused on technical ability and knowledge, rather than in participative democracy focused on shared capabilities in communication. In 2004, we videotaped orthopaedic surgical teams. Analysis revealed a clear and consistent pattern that favoured one-way communication (telling, informing, confronting) over dialogue (asking questions, inviting participation), working against 'assembly' democracy (Keane, 2009).

Co-ordination of care across clinical teams is greatly enhanced by participative democratic structures (Iedema, 2007), sometimes facilitated by objects (artefacts) such as protocols (Gawande, 2009). However, autocratic structures retain a strong, historically contingent presence in medicine and, particularly, surgery. While there is a solid base of evidence suggesting that expanding out to collaboration and connection, rather than shrinking back to the individual, is fundamental to developing a learning organisation (Christakis and Fowler, 2010; Surowiecki, 2005), this again bumps up against a historically contingent ideology in medicine and surgery of heroic individualism – itself grounded in the Protestant ethic of self-help.

Where collaboration is not in the historical grain of surgical practice, it has to be learnt. Ikegami's study of the development of 'aesthetic networks' in feudal Japan (2005) shows that horizontal, shared and democratic practices can develop within historically conditioned autocracies and hierarchies. Mutual interests in art and craft encouraged horizontal social interactions that suspended normal, strict rules of conduct based on vertical social hierarchies. The 'non-technical' or shared elements of surgical work (Flin *et al.*, 2008) – communication, teamwork and aspects of decision-making – can be configured as practice 'artistry' (Bleakley *et al.*, 2011), an aesthetic network of immaterial or emotional labour, binding practices horizontally; while technical practices can be expressed not in terms of autocracies but in terms of meritocracies.

Initiation of a network: champions meet sceptics

In late 2002, we were faced with how we could *initiate* a network through increasing our number of allies, mobilising actors to affect other actors in translations yielding innovation. Enrolment of allies includes negotiating terms of participation, and this forum initiated a key debate about how the entire range of OT personnel could be centrally involved in the project through shared communication and teamwork practices.

We set up an exploratory dialogue between six champions (four consultant anaesthetists, a consultant surgeon and an experienced nurse) and six sceptics (two consultant surgeons, two consultant anaesthetists and two senior nurses) in a 2-day human factors seminar. This initiated a dialogical process, where 'an interventionist research methodology is needed which aims at pushing forward, mediating, recording and analyzing cycles of expansive learning in local activity systems' (Engeström, 2008, p.2). Some key sceptics (surgeons), for example, were persuaded to road test briefing. Others were deeply ambivalent, mistaking research for management surveillance and already threatening to rupture a delicate, nascent network.

Some radical ideas emerged – for example, how nurses or operating department assistants traditionally low on the hierarchy could be empowered to speak out (a form of 'moral courage' but also an act of professionalism) if they saw activity that might jeopardise a patient's safety. The more 'moral courage' was slighted by sceptics (including some nurses) so the network paradoxically strengthened, and moral courage became an actor and key ally in its own right (Bleakley, 2006b).

Funding

Funding is patently a key actor in research, allowing for enrolment of allies. It can, however, act as an intermediary rather than a mediator, supporting a sterile network with lack of translations and a poor net effect, rather than a dynamic network of fertile associations and translations promising innovation, knowledge production and practice change. Funding translates across actors, e.g. buying in the expertise of clinicians to work as researchers.

Grants allowed us, for example, to collaborate with the author of a North American, validated Safety Attitudes Questionnaire (SAQ), in anglicising the SAQ for UK practitioners (Sexton *et al.*, 2006); to buy in a full-time researcher and two PhD students; to buy in expertise to develop team self-review (briefing and debriefing) (Henderson *et al.*, 2007); and to install videotape recording facilities in two OTs, where, once ethical clearance was received, we could record routine work to supplement ethnographic observations. Videotaped extracts were played back to teams as a stimulus to a 'hot' debriefing, offering a major innovation in research methodology and a powerful addition to the overall educational 'interruption' (Bleakley *et al.*, 2004).

While no surgical team members were in any way forced to engage with the project, a few did harden opinion against its value, culminating in an act of defiance (or sabotage) through physically dismantling connecting cables in the video set-up. After 6 months of sporadic filming – gaining key insights – we abandoned the video ethnography to appease the minority of dissenters. By not engaging in open confrontation but accepting the depth of feeling of the clinicians concerned and their rationale for such feeling (suspicion that the project was ultimately a form of management surveillance, questioning surgeons' autonomy), we gained some respect from those clinicians. We followed the advice of Sun Tzu's *The Art of War* that strategy and not hostility wins allies.

Other grants allowed us to do the following.

- Employ an experienced theatre nurse to support and evaluate briefing activities over a period of 6 months (Allard *et al.*, 2007).
- Develop a close-call reporting system that later included hiring a recently retired consultant anaesthetist to close the loop locally on reports, where an issue raised by a report is addressed with practitioners in an effort to resolve the issue (e.g. ensuring that protocols are adhered to, or that faulty equipment is fixed rapidly) (Hobbs and Bleakley, 2005).
- Set up a centre of excellence recognised by European Social Funding as a platform for international networking and to develop the open-access website (www.ttrm.co.uk).

The website offers a mixed blessing through a design fault. While promising to act as an ally in mediating translations between actors, an interactive component was not built in so that the website paradoxically became an intermediary rather than a mediator – a frozen web and repository of authoritative information, rather than a site for translation and negotiation. One of our aims for the near future is to raise funds to develop interactive elements for the website.

A multi-professional conference

In December 2002, we arranged a 1-day human factors symposium for as many staff as possible to advertise and kick-start the project. OTs closed down apart from emergency provision, and attendees ranged from cleaners and porters to consultant surgeons and key members of management and the public, including the chair of the trust. The morning offered unique small-group discussions, where cleaners and porters discussed issues along with researchers, managers and clinicians. Many reported that this was the first time that they had experienced such a democratic levelling. The afternoon offered specialist input from an ex airline pilot turned safety champion and from human factors researchers, including data from observation of paediatric heart surgery teams.

Consciousness raising was clearly established and the network effect was powerful and formative. However, the conference also had the paradoxical effect of producing a kind of toxic shock. While bringing home the message concerning the importance of improving teamworking to establish a patient safety culture, the news from the airlines that such a culture change took around 15 years to establish, produced a kind of numbing among some participants, as if the challenge was actually too great to contemplate.

Hard and soft design

Cumulative, unidirectional attitude change creates a climate and lays the foundation for culture change. We saw no point in attempting to change work activities without first changing attitudes towards that work. This would be equivalent to introducing a mandatory protocol without the will of those who would have to follow it.

Our key outcome measure of climate change was cumulative scores on each component of the SAQ – particularly 'teamwork' and 'safety climate'. Significant positive changes in scores from a baseline measure would indicate a climate shift. We were also – serendipitously – able to offer the intervention to one discrete OT complex and then to a second complex of similar size 1 year later to compare both cumulative SAQ scores across complexes and changes from baseline scores within complexes. To gauge culture change, we employed qualitative methods guided by an ANT framework – ethnographic observations, videotaped examples of practice, open-ended interviews and free-text comments on the SAQ.

In using the SAQ, alliances were made with an international community of researchers, widening the network effect and multiplying the numbers of actors as mediators, again facilitating translations leading to innovations. The author of the SAQ was able to insert our baseline data into an international database, so that we could compare scores from our hospital cohort with those from other OT cohorts internationally. This proved to be effective leverage data in persuading our senior management to become mediating actors in the widening network, where, in comparison with a large number of international hospital cohorts, our SAQ scores indicated a relatively low level of development of an active safety culture as perceived by OT personnel. This one piece of evidence served initially as an effective way to gain senior management allies in strengthening the patient safety work-net/network, although key senior management figures in general have acted as intermediaries rather than mediators in the project.

Team self-review

Having confirmed through observation a lack of a culture of team self-review, a team of social science researchers and clinicians modelled, initiated and facilitated briefing and debriefing practices across a sample of OT teams. A comprehensive handbook of techniques was produced and distilled down to bullet points on credit card-sized prompts circulated to all OT staff (Henderson *et al.*, 2007). Suggested practices encouraged team building through communication, reflective practice (debrief), and reflexive accounting (innovation resulting from team self-review) (Bleakley *et al.*, 2011), cumulatively building a safety net for patients. This was further networked through the key artefact (actor) of a regular newsletter circulated among all OT staff that kept them up to date on research findings and implications, including the percentage of teams carrying out briefing and/or debriefing and accounts of local styles. Data were also fed back and discussed face-to-face at audit and education meetings.

Networking with clinicians and academics

Networks are expanded and strengthened across the clinical education community through dissemination of research texts by publication and conference presentations. Through invitation, we have taken TTRM on the road to many UK hospitals and three Canadian hospitals. Where ANT is still perceived as a radical or even wayward approach within clinical education research and particularly within health services research, where positivistic models dominate, strengthening network effects through creating alliances is an exciting challenge.

Research texts

Texts, such as this chapter, are naturally and sometimes frustratingly partial – but then so is the slice of life that is researched. The point of an ANT approach is to render interesting objects visible that might otherwise remain black-boxed. Visibility of actors and translations between actors is the focus of the research text, re-searching issues through tracing the network.

For example, Frode Heldal (2010) describes complex interactions between members of a breast cancer care team – cytologists, surgeons and radiologists – with emphasis upon key objects, such as X-rays, cytology pictures and a form held by the patient used to record diagnoses and passed among surgeons, cytologists and radiologists as the patient visited each in turn. Heldal followed the breast cancer unit in a Norwegian hospital for 18 months and also conducted interviews, showing how team meetings based around a patient led at best to a 'loosely coupled' system, and at worse to disintegration.

In loosely coupled systems, networks might be traced but were faint and did not stabilise from week to week as the forms of connections between the three specialities were more or less reinvented on every occasion in discussing patients. Tightly coupled systems leading to strong networks were never realised. Potential networks were also frustrated or quickly disintegrated. For example, a radiologist within the team used specialist knowledge to frustrate potential collaboration between specialties by insisting that only radiologists could read X-rays properly. The form held by the patient came to be utilised sequentially by the three specialities, and then acted as an intermediary between those doctors, rather than being used as a mediator in a common meeting. Heldal's account offers a thick description of a potential network that is constantly frustrated, as the inherent potency of objects as mediators (such as the patient's form) is never realised, where such objects, actants or actors only act as intermediaries.

Law (2004, p.21) suggests that ANT research is guided by a baroque rather than a Romantic sensibility, where we should 'look down' to get an overall grasp of relations between actors and the messy, sensuous materiality of practice – detail and texture – rather than looking up for some guiding ideal, a framework or principle. Latour (2007, pp.133–5) suggests keeping a series of notebooks during fieldwork to record the voices of the actors and the effects of translations, the recruitment of allies, your own responses, your wild ideas and the effects of feeding back data to participants.

Public engagement through the arts

The public has come to see medicine and surgery through the rather distorted lens of UK and North American television soap operas (Bleakley *et al.*, 2011). TTRM has widened and strengthened the research network through alliances with dramatists, actors and visual artists in particular to develop public engagement and education projects. These have included schoolchildren making films about their experiences in hospital; visual artists tracking the patients' perspectives from diagnosis through surgery to recovery, presented as video, drawing and painting; and use of actors working with clinicians in scripting and preparation of video vignettes for teaching purposes, also uploaded to the website for open access. The work-net/network effect then also includes the enrolment of web designers. The point of engagement has included gallery exhibitions, public open days and conferences, and the video resources are widely used in teaching medical students and junior doctors. Through medical humanities and medicine and arts funding bodies, these activities have attracted significant research funding.

In summary, the movement into the public arena initiates new actor-network possibilities, where the innovation resulting from translations across the network between actors is the opening to public gaze of what has, historically, been a closed profession.

Work-net/network effects

Rather than list 'outcomes' of the research, an ANT approach would look at the dynamic work-net that has been created. This goes well beyond the immediate instrumental outcomes of research that may be required by a particular funding body, as the earlier section on public engagement illustrates. In ANT, since the outcome of a project depends on the alliances created and the translation effects across an unpredictable number of persons, material objects and ideas, an a priori statement about aims or goals is considered premature. Rather than rational(ised) outcomes, we need to speak of the aggregation of interests determined by the nature of the net effect of the research. Or, what is the quality of impression or trace left by the work-net/network as it is cut at the point of writing up the research work?

What is held primarily as a net effect of the TTRM project so far is a shift in attitudes towards the importance of communication within and across team settings. The cumulative effect of this is the establishment of a safety climate, which we see as the necessary condition of possibility for the emergence of a safety culture – a distinctive change in work practices. Some of this innovation is evident. For example, not only was the ground prepared for the introduction of the World Health Organization's surgical safety checklist but also it is already being translated – *mindfully* utilised within a teambuilding ethos rather than instrumentally, simply as a checklist.

Part III: limitations to actor-network-theory-based research

ANT research demands specialists

By now, some readers will have decided that ANT is not for them – it is perhaps too cavalier; others will find it theory-heavy or simply out of their comfort zone, employing an already idiosyncratic vocabulary idiosyncratically. Others will be attracted to its apparently naïve realism, its refreshing unorthodoxy, its attraction to the problematic, its refusal to offer reductive answers and its radically democratic agenda of generalised symmetry.

ANT sets out pretty stringent conditions for membership. Special qualities are needed for taking ethnography into the territory that ANT delineates, such as sensibilities of witnessing, close noticing and attention to context that are aesthetic and ethical, and not primarily instrumental. Patience and restraint are needed, as fieldwork is intensive and time consuming. Just how such qualities and related identities are developed and performed is not well articulated in the ANT literature. Paradoxically, while ANT proposes a radical democracy of phenomena, it appears to encourage an elite body of researchers.

Key writers such as Bruno Latour and Annemarie Mol are stylists and use experimental forms that set very high standards. Latour in particular takes delight in baroque sentences. Here is a piece of advice for the novice fieldworker concerning translation from notebooks to research text: 'The unique adequacy one should strive for in deploying complex imbroglios cannot be obtained without continuous sketches and draft' (Latour 2007, p.134). Well, 'imbroglio' means entanglement, and surely 'complex' is then redundant? Deployment is a militaristic word meaning to get in place ready for battle and is this really how ANT researchers must go about their business in both fieldwork and writing up? Indeed, ANT's overall stance may look militaristic. This chapter uses similar rhetorical devices – particularly metaphors of 'strengthening' networks and conversely, nascent and delicate networks open to rupture. Perhaps we should use less militaristic tropes, encouraging an ANT sensibility of 'presence' rather than 'force'? For some, the language of force is already gendered male. Perhaps ANT's genesis in science studies rather than the humanities already affords tough-mindedness rather than tender-mindedness.

Can actor-network-theory demand both precision and ambiguity?

ANT seems to demand precision and ambiguity at the same time and this may infect research practices. While Latour (2010, 1993) is at pains to point out that the curse of modernism is to aim for purity (whether through truth seeking or ethnically and racially), where reality is hybrid and messy, what do we make of his insistence on a precise definition of the key notion of 'network', where 'The word network is so ambiguous that we should have abandoned it long ago' (Latour 2007, p.129)? ANT feeds off uncertainties, unexpected turns in events, upsets, slippage in practices, impressions and traces. Surely 'network' must retain ambiguity. As ANT researchers, are we not expected to readily tolerate such ambiguity? Further, in cultivating ambiguity as a virtue, where does morality rest in a network? ANT is strangely silent on the ethics of research.

Does actor-network-theory support animism?

ANT's philosophical position (Harman, 2009) raises the spectre of animism. Where 'actors' include material objects, do objects have agency, and how can interaction between material objects produce non-material effects? ANT's answer to this is straightforward – it does not posit agency for objects, but is interested in the potential and actual connections between things and the outcomes of such connections. As an example, here is a close call report from the operating theatre, part of the dataset of our TTRM study:

> The operating table had a new mattress in place. The patient needed to be positioned naked on a gel mat on the mattress in order to prevent slipping off the table when steep head down tilt is applied to the table. The gel mat was positioned on the table. When the patient was moved onto the gel mat, the gel mat slipped across the table mattress. Because the mattress is very smooth, there is no grip to allow friction between the gel mat and table mattress.

The report does not, however, assign agency to the gel mat or the table mattress. Rather, it points out that the *relationship* between the two is translational or has a transformative effect – of putting the patient at risk through slipping, and then of effecting practice change. Something now has to be done to prevent a reoccurrence. Somebody and some thing has to get a grip. I warned that ANT research is drawn to slippage!

Here is a more serious slippage – one of attention. This report also illustrates the logic of generalised symmetry:

> A valve came loose /detached from a disposable laparoscopic port and into a patient's abdominal cavity. It was only by chance it was noticed inside the patient and then removed.

It is because person, material object and protocol are brought together in translation and mediation in safety-sensitive care that such a scenario would normally never occur. In this case, again, we should suspend thinking about agency for objects and think about connections between things. Indeed connections and disconnections abound, while a main connection was not immediately made – double-checking the patient and the equipment before, during and after procedures so that there is no 'by chance' and a valve does not 'come loose', to ghost in 'by chance'. It is the connection between laparoscope and person that does the work of 'noticing' and picks up on the loose valve, and not the disconnection between person and instrument that is signified in the phrase 'by chance'. But 'chance' is not good enough for optimum patient safety.

Resisting reduction

Finally, and paradoxically, for ANT itself to recruit allies and strengthen its work-net, it must be able to tolerate reduction to its Wikipedia form of presentation (http://en.wikipedia.org/wiki/Actor-network_theory), where it is readily black-boxed, confirming Latour's (1999) fear that a complex apprehension is reduced to a rule of thumb centred on a misunderstanding of 'network'. While

Wikipedia explicitly invites revision, entries appear authoritative, soaked in the ethos of encyclopaedic knowledge and resisting interventions. ANT's Wikipedia entry – strangely spawning a paper equivalent (Anon, 2010) is a good example of a congealed network. The site actually exerts minimum sweat, doing little work where it has settled and crystallised, failing to interact with other actors in a work-net effect of translation. Will ANT's entry over time into clinical education research lead to a similar dilution and congealing of its dynamic concerns, or will it stimulate a welcome revolution in research thinking and method?

References

NB: the items marked * describe the study reported in Part II.

Anon (2010) *Actor-Network Theory*. Memphis, TN, Books LLC.

Akrich, M., Callon, M. and Latour, B. (2002) The key to success in innovation, part I: the art of interessement. *International Journal of Innovation Management*, 6, 187–206.

*Allard, J., Bleakley, A., Hobbs, A., *et al.* (2007) "Who's on the team today?" The status of briefing amongst operating theatre practitioners in one UK hospital. *Journal of Interprofessional Care*, 21(2), 189–206.

*Bleakley, A. (2006a) 'You are who I say you are': the rhetorical construction of identity in the operating theatre. *Journal of Workplace Learning*, 18(7–8), 14–25.

*Bleakley, A. (2006b) A common body of care: the ethics and politics of teamwork in the operating theater are inseparable. *Journal of Medicine and Philosophy*, 31(3), 305–22.

*Bleakley, A., Hobbs, A., Boyden, J., *et al.* (2004) Safety in operating theatres: improving teamwork through team resource management. *Journal of Workplace Learning*, 16(1–2), 83–91.

*Bleakley, A., Boyden, J., Hobbs, A., *et al.* (2006) Improving teamwork climate in operating theatres: the shift from multiprofessionalism to interprofessionalism. *Journal of Interprofessional Care*, 20(5), 461–70.

Bleakley, A., Bligh, J. and Browne, J. (2011) *Medical Education for the Future: identity, power and location*. New York, NY, Springer.

Christakis, N. and Fowler, J. (2010) *Connected: the amazing power of social networks and how they shape our lives*. London, Harper Press.

Engeström, Y. (1999) Learning by expanding: ten years after [introduction to the German edition of *Learning by Expanding*]. Available from: http://lchc.ucsd.edu/MCA/Paper/Engestrom/expanding/intro.htm (accessed 25 January 2012).

Engeström, Y. (2008) *From Teams to Knots*. Cambridge, Cambridge University Press.

Fenwick, T. and Edwards, R. (2010) *Actor-Network Theory in Education*. London, Routledge.

Flin, R., O'Connor, P. and Crichton, M. (2008) *Safety at the Sharp End: a guide to non-technical skills*. Farnham, Surrey, Ashgate.

Gabbay, J. and Le May, A. (2011) *Practice-based Evidence for Healthcare: clinical mind-lines*. London, Routledge.

Garfinkel, H. (1967) *Studies in Ethnomethodology*. Englewood Cliffs, NJ, Prentice-Hall.

Gawande, A. (2009) *The Checklist Manifesto: how to get things right*. London, Profile.

Harman, G. (2009) *Prince of Networks: Bruno Latour and metaphysics*. Melbourne, re.press.

Heldal, F. (2010) Multidisciplinary collaboration as a loosely coupled system: integrating and blocking professional boundaries with objects. *Journal of Interprofessional Care*, 24(1), 19–30.

Henderson, S., Mills M., Hobbs, A. *et al.* (2007) Surgical team self-review: enhancing organisational learning. In: M. Cook, J. Noyes and Y. Masakowski (eds) *Decision Making in Complex Environments*. Aldershot, Ashgate.

Hobbs, A. (2005) Team self-review: improving teamwork and reducing error. *Risk Management: Health Care Risk Report*, 11(6), 16–17.

Hobbs, A. and Bleakley, A. (2005) Close-call reporting. *Risk Management: Health Care Risk Report*, 11(4), 18–19.

Iedema, R. (ed.) (2007) *The Discourse of Hospital Communication: tracing complexities in contemporary health organizations*. Houndsworth, Palgrave Macmillan.

Ikegami, E. (2005) *Bonds of Civility: aesthetic networks and the political origins of Japanese culture*. Cambridge, Cambridge University Press.

Keane, J. (2009) *The Life and Death of Democracy*. New York, NY, Simon & Schuster.

Kohn, L. T., Corrigan, J. M. and Donaldson, M. S. (eds) (1999) *To Err is Human: building a safer health system*. Washington, DC, National Academic Press.

Latour, B. (1993) *We Have Never been Modern*. Hemel Hempstead, Harvester Wheatsheaf.

Latour, B. (1996) *Aramis or the Love of Technology*. Cambridge, MA, Harvard University Press.

Latour B. (1999) On recalling ANT. In: J. Law and J. Hassard (eds) *Actor Network and After*. Oxford, Blackwell, pp.15–25.

Latour, B. (2007) *Reassembling the Social: an introduction to actor-network-theory*. Oxford, Oxford University Press.

Latour, B. (2010) *On the Modern Cult of the Factish Gods*. Durham, NC, Duke University Press.

Law, J. (2004) *After Method: mess in social science research*. London, Routledge.

Law, J. and Singleton, V. (2005) Object lessons. *Organization*, 12(3), 331–55.

Mol, A. (1999) Ontological politics: a word and some questions. In: J. Law and J. Hassard (eds) *Actor Network Theory and After*. Oxford, Blackwell, pp.74–89.

Mol, A. (2002) *The Body Multiple: ontology in medical practice*. Durham, NC, Duke University Press.

Mol, A. (2008) *The Logic of Care: health and the problem of patient choice*. London, Routledge.

Mol, A., Moser, I. and Pols, J (eds) *et al.* (2010) Care: putting practice into theory. In: A. Mol, I. Moser and J. Pols (eds) *Care in Practice: on tinkering in clinics, homes and farms*. Bielefeld, Germany, Transcript-Verlag, pp.7–26.

Pronovost, P. and Vohr, E. (2010) *Safe Patients, Smart Hospitals: how one doctor's checklist can help us change health care from the inside out*. New York, NY, Hudson Street Press.

Schatzki, T. R., Knorr-Cetina, K. and Von Savigny, E. (eds) (2001) *The Practice Turn in Contemporary Theory*. Abingdon, Routledge.

Sexton, J. B., Helmreich, R. L., Neilands, T. B., *et al.* (2006) The Safety Attitudes Questionnaire: psychometric properties, benchmarking data, and emergency research. *BMC Health Services Research*, 6, 44.

Surowiecki, J. (2005) *The Wisdom of Crowds: why the many are smarter than the few*. London, Abacus.

West, M. A. and Borrill, C. S. (2002) *Effective Human Resource Management and Lower Patient Mortality*. Birmingham, University of Aston.

Further reading ...

Callon, M. (1986) Some elements of a sociology of translation: domestication of the scallops and fisherman of St. Brieuc Bay. In: J. Law (ed.) *Power, Action and Belief: a new sociology of knowledge?* London, Routledge.

Edwards, R., Biesta, G. and Thorpe, M. (eds) (2009) *Rethinking Contexts for Learning and Teaching: communities, activities and networks*. London, Routledge.

Latour, B. (1987) *Science in Action: how to follow scientists and engineers through society*. Cambridge, MA, Harvard University Press.

Latour, B. (2004) *Politics of Nature: how to bring the sciences into democracy*. Cambridge, MA, Harvard University Press.

9

Ethnomethodological workplace studies and learning in clinical practice

Will Gibson, Helena Webb and Dirk vom Lehn

WORKPLACE STUDIES IS A BRANCH OF INTERACTIONAL SOCIOLOGY concerned with the analysis of knowledge and practice in work settings. This chapter provides an overview of the key conceptual features of the perspective and an outline of the methodological strategies that are typically applied within it. By drawing on a research study of optometric work practices, the discussion aims to show how this perspective can contribute to the analysis, understanding and design of clinical education. Our analysis of optometric work looks at how problems are established within consultations and at the conduct of a particular eye examination. The interactional practices used by optometrists in these sequences display communication skills that have been learnt in situ rather than through formal education contexts. As assessment relies in many cases on subjective reporting, these communication skills are crucial for establishing accurate evaluations of vision. By producing empirical findings such as those reported in this paper, workplace studies is able to generate important insights that can inform medical educational processes by, for example, preparing trainees to enter clinical professions.

Ethnomethodology and the analysis of work-based learning

Workplace studies is a sociological approach to the analysis of work practices that pays close attention to how people collaborate and co-ordinate their activities in social settings (Luff *et al.*, 2000). The approach is heavily influenced by ethnomethodology (EM) (Garfinkel, 1967), which is a form of social enquiry concerned with the examination of people's methods for producing social life (see Coulon, 1995, for a brief and accessible description of EM). The basic methodological stance of both of these areas of work involves studying, in detail, the common-sense knowledge that people use to make social practices work, paying close attention to the contextual details of real-world actions and the ways in which people go about accomplishing their tasks. 'Common-sense knowledge' is a term Garfinkel (1967) draws from Alfred Schutz (1967), whose phenomenological approach argues for studies that explore how people bring to bear knowledge about the everyday to organise their action in social situations. Workplace studies is also closely linked with EM's 'sister discipline' of conversation analysis (CA; together these studies are often described using the abbreviation EMCA), which shares the concern with the interactional accomplishment of social order, but with a particular focus on the organisation of talk within social action.

The concern with 'common-sense knowledge in action' is seen as important because such knowledge in many ways *constitutes* the activities that people undertake. If we want to understand why social practices take the form that they do – and, indeed, what that form is – then we must know, in detail, what resources people use to make those events occur as they do in the first place. In ethnomethodological studies, this has often involved an examination of apparently 'trivial' aspects of social life, such as queuing behaviour (Watson, 1993), consumption practices in cafés (Laurier *et al.*, 2001), learning kung fu (Girton, 1986) and jazz improvisation (Sudnow, 2001). To give an indication of the type of analysis involved in such studies, Laurier *et al.* (2001) looked closely at the social organisation of a café. This involved exploring the local 'rules' that the people who visited the café used to make sense of the activities being undertaken there, such as seating patterns, table sharing, the ways that tables were laid out, and the signs that people used to demonstrate to others how long they might be staying in the café. The analysis illustrated how users of the café manipulated cutlery, newspapers, chair positions and so on in order to indicate to others that they were variously leaving, about to finish/start eating, not interested in small talk and so on. What we learn from these very detailed examinations of settings is how social life is conducted by participants, and how participants come to produce meanings and intentions within specific social contexts.

Medical work has been a strong area of interest within EMCA and workplace studies (Have, 1995), with empirical investigations of all kinds of settings, including general practitioner consultations (Gibson *et al.*, 2005; Ruusuvuori, 2005; Pilnick, 1998; Heath and Luff, 1996; Greatbatch *et al.*, 1995), accident and emergency rooms (Bjørn and Rødje, 2008; Sbaih, 2002, 1997a, 1997b, 1997c), radiology (Yakel, 2001), nursing (French, 2005; Wakefield *et al.*, 2000, Kelly, 1999; Mason, 1997; Sbaih, 1997a; Bowers, 1992), anaesthesia (Hindmarsh and Pilnick, 2002), pre-hospital care (Greatbatch *et al.*, 2005) and counselling (Peräkylä and Silverman, 1991; Silverman and Peräkylä, 1990). These explorations have helped to demonstrate the local organisation of healthcare practices and the ways that participants in these settings collaboratively organise and negotiate their activities. A strong concern with much of this literature is with the interaction between doctors and patients (see Heath, 1986, and Have, 1995), but also with the role of technology in interaction (Rhodes *et al.*, 2008; Heath and Luff, 2000, 1996; Walther, 1996; Greatbatch *et al.*, 1995), and, more generally, with hospitals as systems of social organisation (Clarke *et al.*, 2006; Sudnow, 1967).

Workplace learning, tacit knowledge and practical action
••••••••••

The empirical focus on work practices within workplace studies produces knowledge about the common-sense, taken-for-granted features of social organisation within particular contexts. This involves showing what participants in the settings need to know in order to operate within those contexts. In doing so, workplace studies can highlight the relationship between training and practice, and show the fit between what people know when they enter a professional work context and what issues they face in learning to operate effectively within it. To give an example related to this project, optometry examinations involve an optometrist and a patient working through a series of tests that are intended to produce an objective assessment of the visual experiences of patients. The tests involve the application of complex technologies such as slit lamps, autorefractors and non-contact tonometers, as well as more mundane tools like eye patches, letter charts and reading stimuli. The various tests in the eye examination are designed to produce a prescription of the patient's vision needs in a way that relies on 'objective' codified categories. Although the examination employs a lot of technical equipment to produce an 'objective' prescription, many of these tests are reliant on input from the patient and the interactions that occur between optometrist and patient to produce the result. Communication skills are therefore vital for the production of optometric consultations. The provision of training in communication processes is increasingly common in optometry courses and textbooks, and many degree programmes have modules that deal with question asking procedures. However, these courses tend to treat communication as a one-way process, and focus on the ways that optometrists ask questions rather than on the interactions between them and patients. There is, then, a potential disjuncture between training and work practices because the skills needed to accomplish the work are not taught prior to the engagement in clinical practice. The study that we describe in this chapter involves an attempt to analyse in detail the organisation of communication practices, and to reflect on the implications for the training of opticians. Although it is not part of the data that we discuss here, a further component of this project entails looking at the ways that optometrists are taught to interact with patients. This gives us an approach to compare these training programmes with real-world communication contexts.

One of the key characteristics of workplace studies is the examination of the very small details of how work is undertaken. In the data discussed here, we look at nuances of speech and body orientation as features of communication. A common complaint about this form of analysis is that researchers in this tradition tend to get obsessed with these details and ignore the broader contexts that inform the work. Indeed, this obsession, it is suggested, actually involves producing a rather strange vision of the work that transforms it into something analytic and removed from the real-world work. However, the methodological orientation stems from an understanding of the character of knowledge and of the relationship between work contexts and learning contexts. It points to the difference between acquiring textbook knowledge and employing such knowledge in the contingent circumstances of actual work settings. A part of learning to become a clinician involves not only learning technical, clinical knowledge, but also learning to apply and to use that knowledge in practice. As Michael Polanyi (1961) famously commented:

> A medical student deepens his [sic] knowledge of a disease by learning a list
> of its symptoms with all their variations, but only clinical practice can teach
> him to integrate the clues observed on an individual patient to form a correct

diagnosis of his illness, rather than an erroneous diagnosis which is often more plausible. (p.460)

The concepts of 'explicit/codified knowledge' and 'tacit knowledge' are often used to help distinguish between skills and forms of knowledge taught in formal education environments (codified knowledge) and those learnt in the workplace (tacit knowledge). One of the key features of tacit knowledge is that it is constituted solely in the work and collaborative practices of those environments. As Gertler (2003) notes, 'much of the tacit knowledge produced within organizations arises "in doing", from the social interaction and collaboration of individual workers within a shared social, organizational, and cultural context' (p.80). In other words, a good deal of the competencies required for a given area of professional practice are learnt through engaging in *the work itself*. Gertler (2003) emphasises that tacit knowledge has a number of key characteristics. First, it exists 'in the background of consciousness' (p.77), as a taken for granted and intuitively known feature of action. Second, and because of this, tacit knowledge is not easily articulated verbally, because 'talking about doing' and 'doing' (or, to use Ryle's (1949) distinction, 'knowing that' and 'knowing how') are distinctive skills. Third, tacit knowledge can only be gained through undertaking the activity to which it pertains, rather than by studying in the abstract. Classic examples of this include activities such as learning to ride a bicycle – the practical skills of balancing while turning peddles and steering handlebars can only be mastered by riding a bicycle. Fourth, the knowledge is, to use Gertler's (2003) language, 'geographically constrained', or in terminology closer to the ethnomethodological perspective, *contextually situated*. As very many studies have shown, each medical setting has its own set of normative characteristics that define the character of *that* work in *that* context.

An important methodological implication of these ideas is that (as a consequence of the first and second points given) studying tacit knowledge may be more productive if it involves looking at what people do, rather than simply *asking people* what they do. Further, (as a consequence of the third and fourth points given) the context of this work is constitutive of the knowledge and practices, and should most logically form a site for its study. The workplace studies approach takes both of these implications seriously as methodological principles. This involves producing a nuanced understanding of the specific operations of knowledge and skills in work contexts. We will move now to discuss the methodology of this approach in further detail.

The methodology of workplace studies

Over the past 20 years or so, workplace studies has arisen as a distinct programme of research that combines the analytic interests of sociologists with the practical concerns of those designing and deploying technology in work settings, such as control rooms of rapid urban transport systems, air traffic control or hospitals. These studies are primarily concerned with understanding the organisational practices of particular work settings and require researchers to gain a detailed insider's view of the ways in which specific contexts operate. Ordinarily, researchers focus on one particular setting (a hospital, ward, practice, surgery and so forth) and apply research methods that uncover the tacit knowledge used by the professionals who work in that setting. In some respects, workplace studies can be described as ethnographic in nature as it shares some important similarities with ethnographic enquiry. Like ethnography, there is an interest in using observations and interviews as forms of fieldwork to gain a rich picture of real-world settings (Delamont, 2007). Equally, workplace studies usually involves data collection for protracted periods. However, there are also some important differences between ethnography and the specific version of ethnomethodological workplace enquiry being described here. Unlike in ethnographic research, the focused interest in this tradition is in the close analysis of video-based data. Transcripts such as those presented in the later sections of this chapter are used to reconstruct in detail the moment-by-moment unfolding processes of interaction. Sections of interaction are selected on the basis of their interest as areas of professional work, and through playing and replaying these sections, detailed transcripts of the talk are made that represent particular features of interest in the talk. Researchers use transcription systems such as that devised by Jefferson (2004) to represent aspects of the interaction that appear relevant to the organisation of the setting. Researchers typically do not try to represent all the features of the interaction, but only those aspects that are regarded as relevant to the analysis. In some instances, researchers also show gestures and gaze as well as talk in such transcripts.

In contrast, ethnography is usually not concerned with interaction as such – and certainly not with its close consideration through video analysis – but with culture, knowledge, custom and social organisation as abstractions (Pollner and Emerson, 2007). Further, in workplace studies, interviews are only used to inform the understanding of the analysis of video observations and not as a means of investigating participants' interpretations of culture. In the study being reported here, conversations with optometrists were necessary in order to make sense of the technical aspects of optometric work, but these interviews were not themselves the area of analysis – rather, they informed our analysis of the transcripts of professional action and interaction. Further, interviews are typically not a good way to tease out issues related to tacit knowledge, because of the difficulties of articulating embodied practice that we highlighted earlier.

Typically, the transcriptions and the videos from which they are produced are used together. As the video is played and replayed, further potentially significant aspects of the interaction are observed and added to the transcript. Transcripts are therefore not static objects, but are changing iterations of particular analytic interest. Analysis very often occurs collaboratively, with teams of researchers working through the data and transcripts together. In the case of the optometry study being discussed in this chapter, optometrists as well as EMCA workplace researchers met regularly to discuss the data and to exchange ideas. A more detailed discussion of the general methodological principles and practices of workplace studies can be found in Heath and Hindmarsh (2002).

In the brief data segments that we present, we wish to explore some basic features of this optometric methodology. One of the aims is to show how the close attention to the real-world activities of healthcare practitioners in specific contexts of their application can show in detail the particular constitutive character of their work. In doing so, it enables us to examine the 'in situ' learning that they acquire as practical skills through these everyday encounters. The context for this discussion is a brief analysis of data relating to the opening section of a consultation and of the distance vision test. We present our data via transcripts of conversations between optometrists and patients. Our analysis shows how information relevant to the consultation is produced through the interactions between optometrist and patient and that the nature of the information produced is contingent on the way those interactions and the consultation more generally are organised by these participants. The processes of constructing a report of vision and eye health that can be used to make prescription decisions are, fundamentally, communicative practices that involve participants defining and constituting problems and perception.

Data analysis

Constructing and defining problems

Standard eye examinations – that is, examinations that have not involved an agreement beforehand between the optometrist and the patient about what the purpose of the consultation is – typically begin with a question from the optometrist that provides the patient with an opportunity to reveal any difficulties he or she is experiencing in connection with his or her eyes. In this section, we focus on some of the basic methodological resources that are frequently used to construct and define those problems.

We start our analysis with the data presented in Figure 9.1 (NB: the transcription system draws on Jefferson's work in conversation analysis. For a discussion of this mode of transcribing, see Have, 2007; Box 9.1 provides a key to the transcription symbols used in our data). The optometrist's question in line 1 comes after the patient has been telling a long anecdote about driving in icy conditions. The question initiates the start of the business of the consultation by seeking an assessment of the patient's eyes and enquires about the existence of problems. This treats the topic of the patient's eyes – and, importantly, the patient's own experience of his eyes – as relevant to the consultation, but does not assume that the patient has had any problems, as the patient may simply be attending for a routine check-up. The issue of 'problems' is not defined by the optometrist in any specific way (e.g. in relation to vision, to eye health, to difficulties with lenses or glasses), but is framed in very general terms, i.e. 'problems with eyes'. The patient responds with a report of an apparent difficulty in seeing ('theh they're ju::st (0.4) sometimes I just can't see fings properly you know?' lines 5–6). The optometrist asks a follow-up question (lines 12–13: 'Do you get it with di:stance things as well? Like signs o:r just with print?). Through this question, the general report of visual problems provided in lines 5 and 6 is treated as being of potential relevance but as requiring further specification. The optometrist's question invokes a key optometric distinction between near and distance vision, which is regularly used within consultations as a basic typology of visual acuity problems. With reference to 'signs' and 'print', the optometrist also provides an example of a type of everyday problem that might count as something within each of these categories. The patient characterises his difficulties in a similarly way by describing the problems he has in reading compact disc covers (lines 17–23).

One of the points that this example helps to show is the way that visual problems need to be identified and categorised through the interaction. The problems are often difficult to formulate, as might be the case in this instance, where the initial presentation of the problem is merely in terms of 'problems with seeing'. One of the roles of the optometrist is to help the patient to describe the problem. Here we see that the distinction of distance and reading, and the reference to real-world contexts of activity are key resources that are used to help do this.

A further point to emphasise in relation to this extract is that this verbal

```
 1. Opt:   .HH How've the eyes been? Have you noticed
 2.        a:ny problems?
 3. Pat:   tchk
 4.        (0.6)
 5. Pat:   The:h they're ju::st (0.4) sometimes I just
 6.        can't see fings properly you know?
 7.        (0.3)
 8. Opt:   Mhm. ptck Is tha:t mo[:re when things
 9. Pat:                         [Like print wise u:n
10. Opt:   ↑O↓kay.
          (0.2)
11. Opt:   Do you get it with di:stance things as
          well? like signs o:r just with [print?
12. Pat:                                  [Na:h
13. Pat:   nah nah. [No I wuh I cun see: (0.3)
14. Opt:            [ºOkayº
15.       o:ka:y, it's just that i:f I wa:s (0.2)
16.       ºptchº say I was in a shop or someing I was
17.       gonna buy a cee dee or someing
18.       like that, I ca::n't, (1.0) I mi:ght be a'le
19.       to see what the grou:p is (name) but I tr:y
20.       un see the: (.) (fing) un I':m I'm just
21.       constantly
22.       (0.3)
```

FIGURE 9.1 Categorising visual problems

exchange occurs while the optometrist makes notes in the electronic patient
record. At the beginning of the section of speech the optometrist is readying the
computer for the consultation (Image 1 in Figure 9.2). He clicks on a textbox on
the screen, making it ready for him to type in information. The bold text under
the images indicates the point of the speech where the picture was taken. The
optometrist keeps his orientation towards the screen until the word 'problems',
where he turns his head and his gaze to the patient who, in turn, shifts his gaze
away from the optometrist into the distance. The optometrist maintains his
hands in a readiness position on the keyboard and keeps looking at the patient
while he delivers his report on his vision. The optometrist holds this gaze and

Box 9.1 Transcription system

(.)	Very brief pause
(0.3)	Specific duration of pause in tenths of a second
[ ]	Overlapping speech
(.h)	Inward breath
:	Elongated sound
_____	Emphasis through louder speech
{ }	Description of non-linguistic behaviour
° °	Quiet speech
Opt	Optometrist speaking
Pat	Patient speaking
><	Quickly spoken talk
↑	Raising intonation

bodily orientation towards the patient until just after asking the patient if he has problems with his distance vision (Figure 9.3), at which point he turns away and begins to enter information into the record.

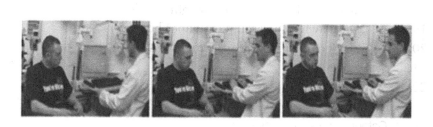

How've the <u>eyes</u> be<u>en</u>?   Have you <u>noticed</u> a:ny **pro**blems?

FIGURE 9.2 Organising note taking and conversational dialogue (note: the authors would like to thank the patient and the optometrist for permission to use these photographs)

The process of taking notes during the consultation is organised around the dialogue. More specifically, the note taking is undertaken in such a way as not to interfere with the spoken interaction. After the interaction represented in Figure 9.2 the optometrist gazes at the patient while he is answering the optometrist's question about his vision (Figure 9.3); he continues to do so throughout his follow-up question and only turns away once the patient has provided his answer.

The patient's 'Na'h nah nah' and the slight pause that follows it and precedes the subsequent 'No', are treated by the optometrist as the possible end of a conversational turn, and an opportunity to shift his gaze and orientation towards the computer and to enter the information (Figure 9.3). The process of transforming the patient's report into recordable information, then, involves the careful use of question-answer sequences, which help the patient to identify relevant information in ways that can be dealt with through the consultation. The recording of this information is managed so that it does not interfere with this reporting process.

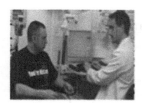 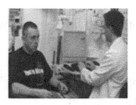

...**with** di:stance things as well like signs o:r just with [print?]
[Na:h nah nah. **No**, I can see

FIGURE 9.3 Entering information into the patient's electronic record (note: the authors would like to thank the patient and the optometrist for permission to use these photographs)

The next fragment helps to illustrate some of these points further. One of the issues related to defining problems is the context in which the consultation sits in relation to the patient's broader treatment history. There are a number of general circumstances that might characterise the context of the visit: patients who visit at regular intermittent intervals for a check-up (as in Figure 9.1); patients who are new members of the practice (who might or might not have a clear problem to address); and patients who attend because they have a particular problem or issue. Optometrists frequently precede their opening questions with a reference to the timing of the patient's last visit. In Figure 9.4, the reference to the patient's visit as 'not too long ago' (line 1 – paraphrase) and 'About November' (line 4 – paraphrase), suggest that the patient has returned earlier than usual. Rather than commenting on the relationship of his visit to this broader history of consultations, the patient adds a description of a new vision problem. He treats the optometrist's reference to time as providing an opportunity to report this, and perhaps even as necessitating it, since the patient could appear to be behaving unreasonably by seeking the optometrist's time so soon. In other words, by reporting that he has some kind of recent problem at the first opportunity, he makes clear that he has a good reason for attending the appointment.

The problem is again defined in quite general terms ('the left e:ye seems to be a lot worse', lines 7–8). The optometrist acknowledges his report in line 9 ('We'll have a look for you:') and in so doing treats it as relevant to the consultation, indicating that exploring it will be an aim within their interaction. The optometrist goes on to ask further questions about the patient's problem (lines 11–12 and line 17). Once again, in these questions the optometrist invokes a distinction between distance and reading, and the patient uses this distinction to provide a further elaboration of the problem.

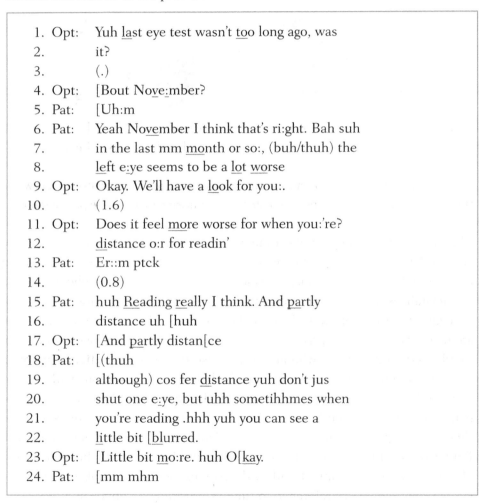

```
 1. Opt:   Yuh last eye test wasn't too long ago, was
 2.        it?
 3.        (.)
 4. Opt:   [Bout Nove:mber?
 5. Pat:   [Uh:m
 6. Pat:   Yeah November I think that's ri:ght. Bah suh
 7.        in the last mm month or so:, (buh/thuh) the
 8.        left e:ye seems to be a lot worse
 9. Opt:   Okay. We'll have a look for you:.
10.        (1.6)
11. Opt:   Does it feel more worse for when you:'re?
12.        distance o:r for readin'
13. Pat:   Er::m ptck
14.        (0.8)
15. Pat:   huh Reading really I think. And partly
16.        distance uh [huh
17. Opt:   [And partly distan[ce
18. Pat:   [(thuh
19.        although) cos fer distance yuh don't jus
20.        shut one e:ye, but uhh sometihhmes when
21.        you're reading .hhh yuh you can see a
22.        little bit [blurred.
23. Opt:   [Little bit mo:re. huh O[kay.
24. Pat:   [mm mhm
```

FIGURE 9.4 Defining the context of the consultation

Through these three short examples we can see a number of key points: identifying and defining possible problems is one of the key aims of the consultation, and figuring out 'what counts as a problem' is a central issue oriented to by both patients and optometrists. Exposing problems is particularly important at the start of the consultation as it sets an agenda for what is to follow. Even though the tests in the standard exam may be the same, the focus of the encounter may change according to whether the patient has expressed concerns or states that he or she just wants a check-up.

Vision problems are not easily categorised and optometrists and patients use the consultation to work together to configure the problematics. The questioning sequences used by the optometrist are critical in this process. We saw that distinctions such as 'reading/distance' are one way in which problems are defined. Similarly, optometrists and patients frequently use real-world contexts as ways of 'trying out' problems, such as reading road signs or instructions on food packets, or seeing other people in the street. The importance of these observations is that the process of testing vision involves identifying problems that form the focus of the test. The test is directed toward solving the problem. Fundamentally, the process of establishing problems is not one that is typically taught to optometrists, but is a professional skill that is learnt through experience. As we noted earlier, textbooks and other training contexts do address the optometrist's conduct and do reflect on the difference between open and closed questions as means of soliciting information. However, the *interaction* between patients and optometrists and the contextual working through of problems is not explored in the curriculum.

In the next section, we look at an example of one of the tests carried out to work through vision problems: the distance vision test. This test is the one that is classically associated with the profession, and is designed to produce an objective score through the use of a wall chart of letters. However, our analysis indicates that the score is highly dependent on the nature of the interaction that surrounds its deployment.

The distance vision test

This is typically the first test in the examination, and usually comes after the opening sequences discussed earlier and some further history taking. The distance vision test is intended to assess the clarity of the patient's vision over distance. With one eye covered, patients are asked to look at a chart of rows of letters that get progressively smaller and read out what they can see. The test produces an 'objective' score based on the size of the letters that patients are able to read correctly. As with the definition of problems however, the test is contingent on the interactions between optometrist and patient.

In Figure 9.5, the optometrist signals the start of the test by instructing the patient where to look at the chart. He then asks whether she can 'see' a line ('>Can you see< the top line there please.', lines 3–4). The patient responds by reading out the letters on the line (line 5). In doing so, she displays that she understands the optometrist's question as an instruction to demonstrate her ability to read the letters (rather than, say, to deliver a general report on whether or not she can). The patient demonstrates a basic competence in understanding how the test is to be carried out, and her role within it. The optometrist treats the patient's reading as an interactional 'turn', and he does not attempt to talk until the patient has finished reading the line of letters. The optometrist provides an 'acknowledgement token' in line 6 ('Excellent') – that is, a speech act that acknowledges that a conversational turn has been taken and, in this case, that it was successfully completed in an appropriate manner. The optometrist continues by directing the patient to read a different line on the chart. This instruction and response sequence forms the basic organisational structure of the distance vision test.

> 1. Opt: Ca::n you see the top line there please?
> 2. Pat: tee ze:d bee eff
> 3. Opt: Ye:ah. >Can you see< the top line there
> 4.   please.
> 5. Pat: ee vee oh tee
> 6. Opt: Excellent looking at the oh on the bottom
> 7.   line the:re,

FIGURE 9.5 Beginning the distance vision test

In the next example (Figure 9.6) we can see the importance of the interactional encounter and of the communication processes within it as resources used for producing a test result. The example starts in a normal way with the optometrist directing the patient to read a line from the chart ('d'you think you can read a:nything on the middle line?', lines 6–7). The patient then proceeds to read out the line (line 9), before being directed by the optometrist to another line of letters (line 10). This basic sequence of request for reading and response by the patient is repeated until no more lines can be read. Within this example, we can see some of the important features of the interactional configuration of test results. Firstly, the optometrist can draw on the ways in which patients read a line as a resource for making a preliminary clinical assessment. A key aspect of this is that the optometrist often treats the silence before a line is read as an indication of difficulty. Although optometrists do not attempt to talk during the reading of a line, they do if there is a substantial pause before the patient begins reading the line. We can see this in the sequence of turns between lines 10 and 13, where the optometrist's request to the patient to read on the bottom line (line 10), is followed by a long pause (line 11), which the optometrist treats as a sign of possible difficulty ('>if you can<', line 12). The same pattern is seen between lines 14 and 21, where the pause (line 16) following the optometrist's request (lines 14–15) is taken as a sign of difficulty in reading ('[might not get very ma:ny]', line 18). In both instances, the optometrist introduces the possibility of failure, providing a warrant for not accomplishing the task by suggesting that it may not be possible. The patient responds to the optometrist's request (in line 15), and his recognition of possible trouble (lines 17–18) by stating that he cannot read the lines ('nnnnnnnnnnnnnnnnnn] no', line 19).

```
 1. Pat:   mm m[hm
 2. Opt:   [Just check your vision, so I'm going
 3.        tuh [cover over this eye he:re,
 4. Pat:             [mm?
 5. Pat:   mm mhm?
 6. Opt:   and d'you think you can read a:nything on the
 7.        middle line?
 8.        (0.2)
 9. Pat:   e::r, (0.6) eFf eN Pee Ee Uu,
10. Opt:   That's grea:t an the bottom one at all?
11.        (1.3)
12. Opt:   >If you can<
13. Pat:   Pee:, (0.6) >aitcH or e:Nn< Dee: whY Zed.
14. Opt:   Great. And a ↑bit↓ of a challenge, but
15.        anything at a::ll on that bo:ttom line?
16.        (0.4)
17. Opt:   You mi:ght not uh got you ver-yea:h
18.        [might not get very ma:ny.]
19. Pat:   [nnnnnnnnnnnnnnnnnnnnnnnnnnn] no
20.        (0.4)
21. Opt:   °Nothing on tha:t.° [So I'll] swa:p that
```

22. Pat: [No]
23. Opt: acro:ss
24.   (.)
25. Opt: agai:n anything on the <u>mi</u>ddle line?
26.   (0.2)
27. Pat: e::r <u>ai</u>tcH ahR <u>Zed</u>
28.   (.)
29. Pat: Ee Pee?
30. Opt: That's ↑it↓ and the <u>bott</u>om one at all?
31.   (0.5)
32. Pat: e::r, (.) a:hR eFf Ee: eM
33.   (0.3)
34. Pat: eN?
35. Opt: <u>E</u>xcellent well <u>do</u>ne. So that's <u>ac</u>tually
36.   a<u>bo</u>:ve average on that <u>bott</u>om li:ne.
37.   [Very goo:d]
38. Pat: [I s it?] o:h ri:ght: yeah

FIGURE 9.6 Interactional features of the distance vision test

An important point to emphasise here is that patients frequently attend to the distance vision test as something they should do 'well', rather than simply as a technical check of the quality of their vision. Optometrists have reported to us that patients often don't try to read lines of letters that they could manage because of a fear of failure. While this is difficult to evidence in the kind of examples provided here, it is clear that optometrists do use methodologies that accommodate failure and try to create an environment in which failure, or partial success, is regarded as an acceptable outcome. This encourages patients to read lines that they might not otherwise attempt. This is important for the diagnosis, as reading some of the letters correctly gives the patient a 'better' score than if they had not attempted any.

Requests to read lines can be made tentatively ('d'you think you can <u>read</u> a:nything on the <u>mi</u>ddle <u>li</u>ne?', lines 6–7: 'an the <u>bott</u>om one at <u>all</u>?', line 10) in order to provide the possibility that failure may occur. Further, optometrists often (although not always) provide a verbal assessment of the patient's reading. Where these assessments occur, they are almost always either neutral or, in the case of the examples provided, positive (i.e. 'that's grea:t', line 10: 'Great', line 14). As we stated earlier, the subjective reporting of visual ability is crucial to the provision of appropriate prescriptions. What the examples illustrate is that the test apparatus (charts and other technical devices) do not create a result, but are merely resources that are used to interactionally establish the limits of vision. The methodology for employing those devices, for working through what counts as a problem and the various tests that define that problem in more detail, is, fundamentally, constituted in communicative competence.

Conclusion: workplace studies and workplace learning

As we suggested earlier, an important conceptual component of workplace studies and related areas of research is that the 'normative' dimensions of the setting in the form of the tacit knowledge of 'how to do such and such' *constitute* and structure the work itself (Suchman, 1996). A very similar point is emphasised by theorists interested in the organisation of learning in workplace contexts, who point to the localised nature of knowledge and know-how (Billett, 2002; Engeström and Middleton, 1996). This has serious implications for the way we understand processes of learning. As Billet (2002) notes, if

> learning is conceptualised more broadly as being the product of participation in social practice … through individuals' engagement in its activities and access to its affordances, it may be possible to adopt a broader view of learning experiences in workplaces and their enhancement. (p.57)

The firm distinction between 'learning environments' and 'work environments' becomes problematic in this view, as the particular features of a given work environment will require the development of context-specific knowledge, which may require workplace training of some kind.

The brief analysis that we provided of optometric practice highlights the importance of communication processes within optometry for achieving a test result. The clinical and technical knowledge related to optometry, and the specialised apparatus that is employed to test eyesight are all used within interactional contexts. The communication processes that organise the test contexts are not a well-developed aspect of optometric training, but are predominantly learnt through experience in practice. Through the analysis that we conduct in this project, and in very close consultation with optometrists, we aim to develop training courses that bridge the gap between work contexts and learning contexts. One of the most important tools used for doing this involves the use of video recordings of optometric consultations. Optometrists have already noted that these tools enable them to become aware of taken for granted areas of work and provides a means for making tacitly learnt actions visible and available for consideration.

The perspective of workplace studies offers an empirical approach for understanding in detail the very specific ways in which tacit knowledge operates in those environments. As we saw earlier, the key characteristics of tacit knowledge are that it operates in the background of consciousness, it is hard to articulate verbally, it is learnt through doing and it is contextual. Therefore, there is a problem for the workplace students in that in addition to the very pragmatic issues of 'getting on' in the setting, they need, in essence, to research the environments so that they can learn how to do the jobs required of them. Workplace studies aims to study these types of environments and to produce findings related to the contextual operation of skills and practices that can inform the design of educational programmes for workers in those environments. In this respect, it offers a very useful methodological approach for those who wish to understand in detail the challenging and changing contexts of medical practice.

Acknowledgements

The data discussed in this chapter come from an Economic and Social Research Council–funded project – RES-062-23-1391 – 'Assessing Eye Sight and Ocular Health: The Practical Work of Optometrists'. We would like to thank the Economic and Social Research Council for its generous support for this research.

References

Billett, S. (2002) Critiquing workplace learning discourses: participation and continuity at work. *Studies in the Education of Adults*, 34(1), 56–67.

Bjørn, P. and Rødje, K. (2008) Triage drift: a workplace study in a pediatric emergency department. *Computer Supported Cooperative Work*, 17(4), 395–419.

Bowers, L. (1992) Ethnomethodology: an approach to nursing research. *International Journal of Nursing Studies*, 29(1), 59–67.

Clarke, K., Hughes, J., Rouncefield, M. and Sommerville, I. (2006) When a bed is not a bed: calculation and calculability in complex organisational settings. In: K. Clarke, G. Hardstone, M. Rouncefield, *et al.* (eds) *Trust in Technology: a socio-technical perspective*. Dordrecht, Springer, pp.21–38.

Coulon, A. (1995) *Ethnomethodology*. London, Sage.

Delamont, S. (2007) Ethnography and participant observation. In: C. Seale, G. Gobo, J. F. Gubrium, *et al.* (eds) *Qualitative Research Practice*. London, Sage, pp.217–29.

Engeström, Y. and Middleton, D. (1996) Introduction: studying work as mindful practice. In: Y. Engeström and D. Middleton (eds) *Cognition and Communication at Work*. Cambridge, Cambridge University Press, pp.1–14.

French, B. (2005) The process of research use in nursing. *Journal of Advanced Nursing*, 49(2), 125–34.

Garfinkel, H. (1967) *Studies in Ethnomethodology*. Englewood Cliffs, NJ, Prentice Hall.

Gertler, M. S. (2003) Tacit knowledge and the economic geography of context, or the undefinable tacitness of being (there). *Journal of Economic Geography*, 3(1), 75–99.

Gibson, M., Jenkings, K. N., Wilson, R., *et al.* (2005) Multi-tasking in practice: coordinated activities in the computer supported doctor-patient consultation. *Medical Informatics*, 74(6), 425–536.

Girton, G. (1986) Kung-fu: towards a praxiological hermeneutic of the martial arts. In: H. Garfinkel (ed.) *Ethnomethodological Studies of Work*. London, Routledge, 60–91.

Greatbatch, D., Heath, C., Campion, P., *et al.* (1995) How do desk-top computers affect the doctor-patient interaction? *Family Practice*, 12(1), 32–6.

Greatbatch, D. G., Hanlon, G., Goode, J., *et al.* (2005) Telephone triage, expert systems and clinical expertise. *Sociology of Health and Illness*, 27(6), 802–30.

Have, P. ten (1995) Medical ethnomethodology: an overview. *Human Studies*, 18(2), 245–61.

Have, P. ten (2007) *Doing Conversation Analysis*. London, Sage.

Heath, C. (1986) *Body Movement and Speech in Medical Interaction*. Cambridge, Cambridge University Press.

Heath, C. and Hindmarsh, J. (2002) Analysing interaction: video, ethnography and situated conduct. In: T. May (ed.) *Qualitative Research in Action*, London, Sage, pp.99–121.

Heath, C. and Luff, P. (1996) Documents and professional practice: 'bad' organisational reasons for 'good' clinical records. In: G. M. Olson, J. S. Olson and M. S. Ackerman (eds) *Proceedings of the 1996 Conference on Computer Supported Cooperative Work*. Boston, MA, ACM Press, pp.354–63.

Heath, C. and Luff, P. (2000) *Technology in Social Interaction*. Cambridge, Cambridge University Press.

Hindmarsh, J. and Pilnick, A. (2002) The tacit order of teamwork: collaboration and embodied conduct in anaesthesia. *Sociological Quarterly*, 43(2), 139–64.

Jefferson, G. (2004) Glossary of transcript symbols with an introduction. In: G. H. Lerner (ed) *Conversation Analysis: studies from the first generation*. Amsterdam, John Benjamins Publishing Company, pp.13–31.

Kelly, R. (1999) Goings-on in a CCU: an ethnomethodological account of things that go on in a routine hand-over. *Nursing in Critical Care*, 4(2), 85–91.

Laurier, E., Whyte, A. and Buckner, K. (2001) An ethnography of a neighbourhood café: informality, table arrangements and background noise. *Journal of Mundane Behaviour*, 2(2), 195–232.

Luff, P., Hindmarsh, J. and Heath, C. (2000) *Workplace Studies: recovering work practice and informing system design.* Cambridge, Cambridge University Press.

Mason, T. (1997) An ethnomethodological analysis of the use of seclusion. *Journal of Advanced Nursing*, 26(4), 780–9.

Peräkylä, A. and Silverman, D. (1991) Owning experience: describing the experience of other persons. *Text – Interdisciplinary Journal for the Study of Discourse*, 11(3), 441–80.

Pilnick, A. (1998) 'Why didn't you say just that?' Dealing with issues of asymmetry, knowledge and competence in the pharmacist/client encounter. *Sociology of Health and Illness*, 20(1), 29–51.

Polanyi, M. (1961) Knowing and being. *Mind*, 70(280), 458–70.

Pollner, M. and Emerson, R. (2007) Ethnomethodology and ethnography. In: P. Atkinson, A. J. Coffey, S. Delamont, *et al.* (eds) *Handbook of Ethnography*. London, Sage, pp.118–35.

Rhodes, P., Small, N., Rowley, E., *et al.* (2008) Electronic medical records in diabetes consultations: participants' gaze as an interactional resource. *Qualitative Health Research*, 18(9), 1247–63.

Ruusuvuori, J. (2005) 'Empathy' and 'sympathy' in action: attending to patients' troubles in Finnish homeopathic and general practice consultations. *Social Psychology Quarterly*, 68(3), 204–22.

Ryle, G. (1949) *The Concept of Mind*. Oxford, Barnes & Noble.

Sbaih, L. C. (1997a) Becoming an A & E nurse. *Accident and Emergency Nursing*, 5(4), 193–7.

Sbaih, L. C. (1997b) The work of accident and emergency nurses: part I. An introduction to the rules. *Accident and Emergency Nursing*, 5(1), 28–33.

Sbaih, L. C. (1997c) The work of accident and emergency nurses: part 2. A & E maxims: making A & E work unique and special. *Accident and Emergency Nursing*, 5(2), 81–7.

Sbaih, L. C. (2002) Meanings of immediate: the practical use of the Patient's Charter in the accident and emergency department. *Social Science and Medicine*, 54(9), 1345–55.

Schutz, A. (1967) *Collected Essays, Vol. 1.* The Hague, Martinus Nijhoff.

Silverman, D. and Peräkylä, A. (1990) AIDS counselling: the interactional organisation of talk about 'delicate' issues. *Sociology of Health and Illness*, 12(3), 293–318.

Suchman, L. (1996) Constituting shared workspaces. In: Y. Engeström and D. Middleton (eds) *Cognition and Communication at Work*. Cambridge, Cambridge University Press, pp.35–60.

Sudnow, D. (1967) *Passing On: the social organization of dying*. Englewood Cliffs, NJ, Prentice Hall.

Sudnow, D. (2001) *Ways of the Hand: a rewritten account*. Cambridge, MA, MIT Press.

Wakefield, A. (2000). Tensions experienced by student nurses in a changed NHS culture. *Nurse Education Today*, 20(7), 571–8.

Walther, J. B. (1996) Computer-mediated communication: impersonal, interpersonal, and hyperpersonal interaction. *Communication Research*, 23(1), 3–43.

Watson, R. (1993) Fear and loathing on West 42nd Street: a response to William Kornblum's account of Times Square. In: J. R. E. Lee and D. R. Watson (eds) *Final*

Report 'Plan Urbain' Interaction in Public Space. Manchester, Department of Sociology, Manchester University, pp.1–26.

Yakel, E. (2001) The social construction of accountability: radiologists and their record-keeping practices. *Information Society: An International Journal*, 17(4), 233–45.

10

Narrative methodology

Understanding learning experiences in an online programme of professional development

Caroline Daly

Introduction
••••••••••••••••••

Until recently (Conole *et al.*, 2008; Creanor *et al.*, 2006), the contribution of narrative methodology to understanding learning experiences of professionals in online learning contexts has been neglected. This is despite established interest in narrative methods within medical practitioner development (Greenhalgh, 2006; Greenhalgh *et al.*, 2005; Greenhalgh and Hurwitz, 1999), based on the conviction, borrowed from research in the social sciences, that such methods have the flexibility that is necessary to capture and record the complexities of human experiential phenomena (Elliott, 2005; Czarniawska, 2004). Cortazzi (2001) has argued that narrative can enable understanding of learning experiences from the perspectives of the learner, the researcher and/or the medical educator. For the learner, constructing narratives about their experiences is a way to

> organise and interpret experience and communicate it memorably in social contexts. In several ways, narratives make sense and give coherence to our personal and professional lives. (Cortazzi, 2001, p.1)

Thus learners' narratives provide accounts in which they organise their experience to make it meaningful to them and communicable and comprehensible to others in dialogic contexts. For the researcher, 'narrative analysis can offer particular insights and challenges regarding concepts of context, interviewing, participants' accounts, representations of meaning, and performance in research' and is particularly applicable to 'the construction and representation of experience and development' (Cortazzi, 2001).

The following extract from an interview with Lisa describes her experiences of learning on a fully online MSc in primary healthcare, which she is studying part-time to further her professional development. What is this story about? What makes it a 'narrative' from which we can learn about Lisa's professional development (and her peers')?

> It is certainly way different from when I was in university back in the seventies. I find it is much more collaborative and we are kind of building knowledge together. There is always somebody online every day, several times a day, [so] that it is very conducive to building learning. Do you see what I mean? To the point where I really look forward to logging on in the morning to see what has been posted, and who said what. And I find myself thinking – I wonder what so and so would think of this? Because you get to know people's styles of thinking, and what they think, and their point of view and all that. (Narrative interview, Lisa)

We are presented with a range of possibilities when thinking about what this story means. We might interpret it as a story about lifelong learning – she started studying in the seventies, she says. Is it therefore mostly of interest in relation to her personal growth as a professional who has embraced technology and now enjoys 'way different' forms of learning? Is it her story of becoming familiar with contemporary educational thinking and terminology, showing that she can talk confidently about 'building knowledge together'? Is her story changed by being constructed via a telephone interview? Whose story is it anyway, once we start making claims about what it 'means'? It could be about a number of things – it depends. It depends on the research focus of course, but crucially, it also depends on the autobiographical interests of the teller and the subjective perspectives brought to it by those who will analyse the story and render it meaningful in a research context. Certain questions have been decided upon as worth investigating, while others may not be considered so relevant or interesting, for now. Lisa has chosen certain details in recounting her experiences, while others have been omitted or relegated as less personally important or relevant to tell. The *meaning* depends on several acts of interpretation – one being that undertaken by the narrator in order to reconstruct her remembered experiences in order to understand and reflect on them; another being the co-construction of the story so that it makes shared sense between teller and listener in the communicative context of an interview; and a further one developed later by the researcher around the story which has been told, giving it coherence and significance which may or may not have been the same as that intended by the teller. All of these acts of interpretation take place within socio-cultural contexts – stories have to make sense according to our understandings of how the world works and how social beings might act and react within that world.

Programmes which support professional development for medical and clinical practitioners are examples of highly complex socio-cultural contexts in which narrative is one way of enabling us to understand the learning processes and participatory practices of those involved. The learner's experience of engaging with such programmes has an impact on the kind of transformations that take place – in terms of knowledge, skills and an individual's sense of professional identity and capability. Narrative methodology enables us to understand these experiences of engagement for busy practitioners who undertake professional learning alongside their work roles. Complex experiential phenomena occur within socio-cultural contexts for professional learning, such phenomena being, for example, encounters between practitioners and patients, teachers and peers and peer-to-peer interaction in a variety of sites – clinical settings, teaching settings and online professional learning communities.

This chapter considers narrative methodology as acts of interpretation, and explores its potential as a way of investigating and understanding highly complex social phenomena. The chapter will explore how engaging with narrative as a *concept* and as a *methodology* can both advance our understanding of learners' experiences in such contexts and deepen participants' experiential awareness of themselves as learners. Part II illustrates the use of a narrative methodological approach in a study to investigate the learning experiences of participants in an online international masters programme for primary healthcare practitioners.

Part I: conceptualising narrative and narrative methodology

'Narrative' needs to be understood both in broad conceptual terms and in its related methodology in order to recognise how it can contribute to understanding complex human experience. Conceptually, 'narrative' suggests a way of thinking about the nature of human knowledge and how humans are able to make sense of experience in order to understand it and learn from it. Further, narrative is a methodological approach that enables researchers to investigate human experience within socio-cultural contexts. Both conceptually and methodologically, narrative makes it possible to think about professional learning as formed by meaning-making processes that are based on articulating autobiographical and subjective perspectives on events and the associated interactions that take place among participants:

> In logic and in science you attempt to mean what you say. In narrative, to be successful, you mean more than you say and treat a text or utterance as open to interpretation rather than literally fixed with, so to speak, the "truth in the text". (Bruner, 1985, p.109)

The significance for narrative research of what is said lies in its expansive meaning, which is rendered by interpretation. Narrative is thus both an epistemology, a way of thinking about and practising research, and an ontology, a 'habitus', or way of being as an educator, practitioner and researcher. Narrative as an epistemology, or way of 'seeing the world', is rooted in Bruner's (1985) work on 'the meaning of experience' and his arguments for 'believability' that is based on experience. He argues that narrative is a 'mode of thought' – that is, a way of knowing, of understanding, that is based on our ordering of experience or 'filtering' of the world as we encounter it. Narrative seeks explanations of the world, or ways of understanding, rooted in the contexts in which events occur. Such contexts are particular to time and place, and thus offer ways of 'knowing' that are different from attempts to establish constant logico-scientific and empirical 'truth'.

Bruner is interested rather in 'verisimilitude' or 'truth-likeness' in the narratives that individuals construct to organise their experiences in order to make sense of them. The sense – or meaning – of such a narrative is rooted in its 'believability' rather than the absolute authenticity of events. Factual accuracy is less important than the understandings that are derived from engaging with the narrative. Narratives constructed by learners to articulate their experience (through interviews, journals or blogs, for example) can contain internal contradictions and inconsistencies. As such, enquirers do not set out to interpret the 'truth' of what participants tell as an accurate representation of the reality of what has happened. Rather, they are interested in what Bruner (1993) claims individuals can come to know, think and feel through their engagement in the 'landscape of consciousness'.

Concepts based on narrative *function* are arguably most relevant to researching professional learning contexts, as these provide a way for narrative to act as a key way of understanding meaning-making processes and the production of professional identities, as defined by Polkinghorne (1988, p.1):

> Narrative meaning is a cognitive process that organizes human experiences into temporarily meaningful episodes. Because this is a cognitive process, a mental operation, narrative meaning is not an 'object' available to direct observation. However, the individual stories and histories that emerge in the creation of human narratives are available for direct observation. Examples of narrative include … the everyday stories we use to explain our own and other's actions.

Narrative *function* focuses on the ways in which the organisation of experience deepens self-awareness and can therefore play a role in the critical review of the professional self, affecting professional identity. This is what distinguishes insights gained from narrative methodology's focus on 'telling'. Eliciting 'telling' is central to narrative research. Different participants' accounts provide alternative or multiple versions of reality, which may challenge superficial, unified, grand narrative and/or 'common sense' versions of professional identity and practice. For example, an experienced general practitioner (GP) sends confident and well-informed electronic postings to her online discussion group as part of her masters programme; then, in a narrative interview, she tells of how she 'feels slightly sick' with anxiety whenever she logs on to begin the next online task with her group. The account given of her learning experiences within a research context contradicts the portrayal of her professional persona online, as constructed in her electronic messages.

Blake (2000, p.194) suggests that the ways in which participants present themselves in online contexts are effectively 'performances', as learners exercise increased power over self-disclosure in a distance situation and create a narrative of how they wish to be seen. Learners are argued to be constantly negotiating their professional and personal identities as they participate in discussing their views and their practice in online learning discussion groups. In narrative research, the GP's 'experience of the experience' is fundamental to deepening our understanding of this relatively new form of professional learning – and also to her own exploration of what is happening here and how she perceives herself as a learner in this medium. Why is it so daunting to present ideas about professional practice in this context? Is it equally difficult for all participants? Is there a gender factor in who feels more or less secure in this environment? What are the sources of anxiety and do they matter for those who design online programmes like this? Narratives of experience as data invite us to ask questions like these, and interpreting them offers challenges to accepted norms or assumptions about professional identity and learning as part of that identity.

Clandinin and Connelly (2000) have identified a clash between what we learn from individual, experiential narratives and the overarching, orthodox version of universal truth, which was described by Lyotard as the 'grand narrative' (1984). Individual experiences of the world might run counter to the official 'story' of how things are. They argue that the grand narrative offers a story about the world in which there is only one version of an issue or an outcome – in this case, one acceptable, unified, confident professional identity available to medical practitioners in how they present themselves and their 'knowledge'. When the grand narratives are challenged by individual narratives which are less certain, we begin to explore in detail the complexity of social phenomena, such as professional learning, and also how individual narratives are positioned in relation to grand narratives which shape, for example, expectations about being and learning as professionals.

The types of questions asked in the earlier paragraphs reflect what Decortis (2004) has called a 'constructivist' approach to working with narrative data. There is a considerable range of perspectives on different forms of narratives as data, and 'constructivist' is one of five main approaches identified by Decortis. This constructivist approach enables us to draw on a 'social orientation' in narrative analysis identified by Bamberg (1997), as opposed to an individual orientation (using narrative as a form of understanding an individual's processes of meaning making within cognitive development). By treating narrative data from a perspective of 'social orientation', we focus on the engagement between individuals and their world:

> [T]he social matrix against which the particular experience is understandable and makes sense is what gives meaning to texts, to accounts of an experience, to the experience itself, and ultimately to the person who is telling it. (p.90)

Narratives can, according to Decortis, be identified as accounts of any type that form a meaningful whole, by which participants create a projection of their experience, either by recounting an episode or presenting a view of something which happened from a perspective that includes or implies other social actors. Thus, some can be lengthy episodes recounting a learning experience, while others may be single sentences which encapsulate a meaningful distillation of a view or perception which the participants offer to make it understandable within the context of an interview or online posting. The approach can be applied to a broad range of types of narrative:

> Third-person and first-person narratives are given equal weight. Explanatory accounts are defined as narratives 'as long as generalised actors (one, you, they) act and position themselves in their actions vis-à-vis others'. (Decortis, 2004, p.7, citing Bamberg, 1997)

Narrative methods involve more than 'logging' experience. They involve capturing, articulating and communicating experience – crucially, the 'experience of the experience' is altered by revisiting it and making it shareable with others (Clandinin and Connelly, 2000). In the example explored next, of researching an online professional learning community, participants were invited to articulate how they learnt with their peers within new technological contexts, and what perceived impact this had on how they developed professional knowledge, attitudes and identities.

Whatever the aims of particular courses, there is evidence that considerable learning is going on which is not course specific or content oriented (Daly *et al.*, 2007; Sharples, 2007; Levy, 2006) but which affects self-concept as learners adapt to collaborative, e-facilitated environments. For the participant, engaging with narrative methods requires that they reflect on their experience of learning within contexts of continual change. Through the research process, educational encounters are revisited and interpreted, so that individual learners are encouraged to develop deeper consideration of their learning and how they have behaved as a learner. Articulating experience encourages participants to consider how relations of various types have helped to constitute their learning: relations with other online learners and tutors whom they may never or rarely meet, with whom they share in the collaborative construction of knowledge in online discussion tasks; and relations with online content of various sorts that offer multiple possibilities for individual searching and presentation of ideas. Such social and technological activity can prompt the participants – once given the opportunity to 'tell' – to reflect on knowledge-building processes that are routinely hidden or subconscious.

The challenges for analysis involve addressing the 'believability' of narrative as data, and the validity of qualitative interpretation of narrative texts. In adopting a narrative approach to the analysis of interview transcripts, journals or electronic postings to an online forum, an interpretive stance is based on hermeneutics, helpfully described by Brown and Dowling (1998) in the claim that all texts are 'an instance of something else'. The challenge is to develop a rationale by which to interpret what that 'something else' might be, and in what circumstances. Essentially, engaging with narrative is a constructivist activity, by which both participant and researcher engage in making sense of the experience – there is no pure, correct 'meaning' to be discovered at any stage. The value of what is 'found' from a constructivist, 'social orientation' perspective, lies in how all involved in the process have deepened their understanding of what has been experienced.

Bamberg's (1997) emphasis on a 'social orientation' in conducting narrative analysis prioritises understanding the experiences and the self, rather than obtaining knowledge and information. Eagleton (2003) argues that it is possible to interpret in such textual contexts, because 'reflecting critically on our situation is part of our situation. It is a feature of the peculiar way we belong to the world ... You do not have to be standing in metaphysical outer-space' (pp.60–2). He argues that all social and human phenomena are open to interpretation, and there is no value in seeking an 'extra-cultural' explanation because it would not be valid anyway:

> To be exact, interpretation must be creative. It must draw upon tacit understandings of how life and language work, practical know-how which can never be precisely formulated ... if we want to be as clear as possible, a certain roughness is unavoidable. (p.206)

This kind of self-awareness is vital to acts of interpretation in narrative research. Thus, narrative analysis sets out to tell the 'story' of the data *according to the researcher's perspective* (which may be different from that of the original teller). How is this perspective to be explicit or open to discussion? Greenhalgh (2006, pp.9–12) has proposed five core criteria for a 'good story' in narrative research, which help to address this challenge, and which help to establish what is meant in practice by Bruner's concept of 'believability' in ascertaining what makes a narrative valuable.

- *Aesthetic appeal*: the narrative is pleasing to hear and recount; it contains an internal harmony.
- *Coherence*: the narrative is clear and makes a logical whole; it contains a 'moral order' or sense.
- *Authenticity*: the narrative has credibility, based on the experiences of the listeners/readers.
- *Reportability*: 'the "so what" value' of what is narrated; its significance.
- *Persuasiveness*: the narrative is convincing in its rendering of the teller's own perspective.

Part II: working with narrative methodology

Narrative methodology was used in a research project that examined the subjective and perceptual experiences of learners in a well-established, fully online, international masters programme in primary healthcare. The participants studied part-time while working in primary healthcare settings around the world. The tutor team described the programme as 'aimed primarily at senior clinicians, researchers, policy makers and leaders in education, with graduates making a significant contribution to primary care development and the establishment of infrastructures for research and teaching programmes in their own countries and regions' (Boynton *et al.*, 2005). Therefore, it was assumed that participants would be used to the concept of collaboration and drawing on experience as a basis for professional learning at masters level. The teaching approach used a co-constructivist design, drawing on experiential learning by which the participants regularly contribute to 'virtual seminars' to learn from one another's experiences in diverse workplaces.

Such e-learning contexts can be characterised as having a flat learning structure, with democratic learning roles in which all participants are actively engaged in constructing professional knowledge. The methods of assessment also encouraged an inductive engagement with ideas. Thus participants drew on critical reflection on work-based experience as a prime source of learning. This involved constructing and sharing experiences, views and interpretations of events and related literature. This kind of approach can of course be highly disorienting for practitioners whose prior experience of medical or clinical education has consisted mainly of individual, cognitive-focused transmission-based learning activities and hierarchical tutor–learner relationships. The online learning model in this programme challenged transmission-mode concepts and traditional orthodoxies about expertise, experience and authoritative knowledge.

However, the research focused not on the features of online pedagogical design but, rather, on the learning experiences of the participants located within this particular programme as a socio-cultural context. Levy (2006) has argued that, in a new relationship between tutors and learners, a focus on learning processes is a major area for future change. Historically, course development in such contexts prioritised the need to develop e-content, learn about student accessibility and participation via different technological tools, and the design of tasks to ensure that learning objectives could be met. New e-learning models such as those used in the programme investigated here involved students in actively constructing their learning in collaborative ways in online discussion fora (Sharples, 2007; McConnell, 2006) and in taking ownership of learning processes (Hall, 2008) by controlling the timing and location of engagement and using online 'persona'. Such contexts have seen a move away from resource-intense, curriculum-focused learning environments, with shifts in responsibility to the learners who co-construct shared understandings of professional phenomena, based on interrogating and interpreting their own experiences.

Sharpe *et al.* (2005) argue that we need more relevant research methodologies to understand what is really happening in these new contexts so that we can better understand learners' experiences. This necessitates the use of research methodologies that focus on the collection of rich qualitative data that capture the learner voice. It can be argued that narrative is one such methodology. In the study of primary healthcare practitioners, narrative methods were used to enable the participants to articulate experiences and 'make sense' of them via sustained, reflective accounts. Methods for eliciting these accounts were conducted at a distance, and thus involved adapting approaches from face-to-face research contexts. The methods used were as follows.

Group narratives: this was a collection of messages posted in response to online tasks at the start of the course, where participants were invited to reflect on their prior learning experiences and expectations on returning to study. Messages were sent within a time frame allowing the participants to work to their own timelines. Participants were inducted into narrative practices requiring them to post their accounts and views, and then respond to each other's postings. Thus they began to establish shared dialogic practices which played a key part in their learning, as described in Greenhalgh (2006), where 'intra-group discussion about what a particular story *means* fuels the learning cycle' (p.40). The process was essentially one of *active* engagement in the evaluation of experiences, and was driven by the learners' priorities, the possibilities of 'different endings' to their stories once they were shared with others, and peer augmentation of the narratives so that new understandings were made possible for all involved. The stories thus became shared social material for their learning.

Telephone interviews: a researcher conducted telephone interviews of 30 minutes with each participant, based on adapting 'postmodern' interviewing (Gubrium, 2003), by which a sustainable narrative flow is facilitated by the interviewer, who makes minimal intervention in respondents' accounts of their experiences. Postmodern interviews are essentially conversations in which the format is constructed within the interview. The emphasis was on giving the participants the opportunity to offer *their* account of their experiences on their own terms. They chose the time of the telephone call and the location to be interviewed, in an attempt to minimise the power differential between the interviewer and interviewee. The postmodern interview provides opportunities for respondent 'emplotment' and 'chronology', which are recognised as key to eliciting personal stories of experience (Greenhalgh *et al.* 2005, p.444). The researcher who conducted individual interviews was not a healthcare practitioner and had never participated in a formal e-learning programme. Therefore the researcher could adopt a genuinely naïve position in relation to the content of interest, thus maximising the need for the respondents to craft their experiences into meaningful narratives. Generic, open questions were used to move the participants to talk about their experiences 'without over-specifying the substance or the perspective of the talk' (McCracken, 1988, p.34).

Online participant commentaries: these have much in common with the narrative interview in terms of facilitating emplotment and rhetorical cohesion but minimise the interviewer–interviewee dynamic. The tutor posted an 'issue' online periodically (e.g. asking for participants' views on how possible they were finding it to form an online 'community'), and they were invited to respond on a voluntary basis. These issues were chosen to explore Luckin *et al.*'s (2001) argument that e-learning can be fragmentary, and experiences may not mirror the coherence intended or presumed within course design.

The online narrative data were produced through the programme's text-based virtual learning environment, and the telephone interviews were transcribed. These data were already a *recontextualised* (Brown and Dowling, 1998) version of actual experiences, because the participants had developed *coherence* by imposing a framework on events and reflections, foregrounding some items while omitting others to 'make sense' of their experiences as part of achieving an effective narrative to communicate. This coherence was constructed – it does not tell us an essential truth about the phenomenon itself. Thus the interview transcripts and online accounts were already different from the actual experiences they reported. How the participants constructed their narrative was in itself of interest. Differences in construction may reflect differences in the participants' own contextual understanding of the discourses of practising primary healthcare, learning and professionalism on which they drew, as well as the research context itself. Practising narrative methodology in itself altered meanings and the significance of events. The experiences themselves had already passed into the participants' history, and so were remembered and articulated from a stance that had already been changed and affected by experience.

By encouraging the participants to narrate 'without over-specifying the substance' (McCracken, 1988, p.34) of the talk, the practitioners elaborated in highly individual ways on their experiences of learning within their online community. Clandinin and Connelly's work (2000) on interpreting narratives highlights the importance of 'maintaining wakefulness' in noting and interrogating the deeper significance of individuals' stories, emphasising that in narrative, meanings are not fixed and are dependent on the context. For all of the participants, learning in a fully online context was new and brought challenges in balancing work–life commitments while studying. It also brought about a re-evaluation of the sources of professional learning and the part they played in one another's development, despite the fact they had never met. The following extract from a narrative interview is an example of Bethan's use of the concept of 'expertise' to convey her interpretation of what has been happening – her own creative meaning making prompts her use of analogy in the context of the interview:

> I think collaboration is a good way to describe it, and just to clarify what I mean, is that it is kind of the way I view the patient doctor interaction, in that everybody in that interaction is an expert in something, and you have got to be respectful of that expertise. And the patient is an expert in their life, and I am more of an expert, somewhat of an expert, in general medicine, and I think that is how it works in the course, where the tutors are experts in the practicalities of the course and what they expect, and what sorts of directions, in general, they want us to go in. But each individual contributor is an expert in the field they work in. And I get the impression that tutors are trying to

glean information, the fact that it is an international course means that they are actually trying to extract information from us, as well, to enrich the course. And I get that feeling very strongly. (Narrative interview, Bethan)

Using an analogy based on 'expertise' like this 'to clarify what I mean' is a strategy frequently used by participants to achieve a shared understanding with the researcher. Bethan interpreted the relationship between the tutors and her fellow learners as distinctly democratic, by which tutors as well as students were learners, and in which the substance of the course was comprised of what the practitioners contributed. This experience led participants to question hierarchical knowledge structures and placed considerable responsibilities on participants to be involved in the learning of their unseen peers. Therefore, there were implications for how the participants perceived professional knowledge and learning. Andy, who worked in a hospital in South Africa, illustrated this when he acknowledged that the diverse professional contexts meant that peer experiences were not directly transferable. He suggested, however, that these differences stimulated other forms of learning:

> We really are rural here, so it is good to hear different opinions, even just from colleagues at nearby hospitals, but to have the opportunity to do that with people from literally completely different settings – in our group, as you know, probably, there are GPs in Canada and orthotics people in Norway and GPs in Pakistan and volunteers in India. It is great to have the different perspectives, not just of different people, but people who are working in, often very different environments, but often surprisingly similar environments, despite being on the other side of the world. And I must say I have really enjoyed that part of it, yeah. And I think, often, sometimes the experience, per se that they have described, isn't necessarily applicable, but it is just so good to have different insights and to remember that the challenges we face and the medicine that we practice has got such a universal application in many ways, and we just have different problems that we have to approach, often quite creatively. And one of the things is just the intellectual stimulation, really, of being forced to think about different things. And combining that with the input that comes from that variety of settings and the variety of students that there are. (Narrative interview, Andy)

This assertion that it is 'just the intellectual stimulation really' could be considered provocative in the context of professional education. He seemed to be asserting that valuable professional growth took place by having certain types of learning relationships with others – regardless of whether what was learnt could be practically applied. His focus on gaining insights, understanding challenges and 'being forced to think about different things' indicated his engagement with transformational and attitudinal aspects of professional development.

The 'believability' of these narratives can be assessed using Greenhalgh's (2006) criteria. It can be argued that both Bethan and Andy narrated aesthetically pleasing accounts – they are coherent, with internal harmonies that follow a coherent train of thought concerning relevant and vivid insights into their experiences. They 'make sense' thematically as accounts centred on learning with peers in online discussion groups. There is ample evidence of authenticity, derived from individual local details of 'being rural here' or noticing that the tutors are 'gleaning information', as well as the personal reflective qualities embedded in both. Both narratives contain significance or 'reportability' for those who want to understand the nature of learning for professionals in online collaborative groups – which is especially relevant in contemporary contexts of considerable growth in e-learning. Finally, the narratives are 'persuasive', in that both narrators convince that they have experienced a co-constructive learning environment, and that this has made an impact on their views of learning. The narrators show a considerable degree of interest in how they learn with others and there is commitment to the collaborative processes.

When the narratives were shared with the course tutors, much of the content did not surprise them – they knew their students well. But the accounts also included counter-narratives that did not normally feature in 'grand narratives' of practitioners who were successful learners. They offered insights that went beyond the information yielded in 'student satisfaction' evaluation data or institutional course exit surveys (Prosser, 2005; Richardson, 2005). The data revealed the ways in which they recalled experiences in ways not anticipated by tutors (e.g. the GP who described 'feeling sick' before posting to the forum; the sheer scale of the struggle to balance work, life and study; the fact that, as students, they participated online in the middle of the working day, e.g. 'between patients'). The narratives also highlighted the need for more close engagement by programme staff with students' experiences and students' desires to 'own' evaluation processes, to decide when and how it was convenient and valuable to discuss their experiences.

The learners' accounts and the tutor responses also illustrate how engaging with narrative in professional learning contexts provoked 'meta-learning'. The participants began to reflect on the learning processes they experienced and projected explanations on to what had happened within the online community.

Narrative methods can enable participants and tutors as well as researchers to participate in interpreting their own orientation to their learning, to further understand their roles as peer learners and to consider how professional formation is brought about by interaction between peers in a diverse range of socio-cultural contexts. Engaging with narrative affects participants' identities as learners. By narrating, these learners learn to examine the contemporary social and technological resources they work with at a meta level. The need for a focus on meta-learning in learning environments supported by technologies has been highlighted by Levy (2006), who suggests that development within the 'process' domain of knowledge (learning to learn) impacts positively on e-learners' progress within the subject or content domain.

Conclusion: are we feeling comfortable?

Narrative is a stance or 'habitus' as a research methodology, by which those involved share a social orientation to the way meanings are made and the value of meaning-making processes. When this is applied to a professional learning context, boundaries become blurred as participants blend the roles of learner, practitioner, narrator or member of the public going about daily life (one doctor related details about her learning experiences via a mobile phone while travelling on a train). Autobiographical perspectives and multifaceted engagement with the world are vital to narrating and interpreting learning experiences. Participants are usually eager narrators and their stories provide rich material for interpretation – what is 'going on' when a new narrative interrupts the one already being told by a doctor in an understaffed accident and emergency hospital department in South Africa, when he stops the telephone interview he has arranged so that he can 'make an incision'? Further rich, complex and sometimes perturbing possibilities are introduced for understanding his professional world and the challenges of learning and practising within it. Our understanding of diverse learners' experiences can be advanced by the multiple acts of interpretation that are brought to narratives, both from those interpretations that carefully capture and reflect on experiences and from those constructed 'on the fly' within the research process itself. We can never be certain about what a story means – but acts of interpretation demand that we explore the 'believability' of the narrator's rendering of experience, and thereby test our own ways of seeing the world. If we are not comfortable with roughness, creativity and a commitment to 'truth-likeness', then narrative research will be frustrating. However, if we are comfortable with narrative as all these things – as a 'mode of thought' – then its relevance to contemporary professional learning contexts is rich with research possibilities.

Acknowledgements

The Centre for Distance Education, University of London, and the Centre for Excellence in Work-based Learning for Education Professionals, Institute of Education, University of London, funded this project. With thanks to the MSc team in Primary Health Care at University College Hospital.

References

Bamberg, M. (1997) *Narrative Development: six approaches*. London, Lawrence Erlbaum.

Blake, N. (2000) Tutors and students without faces or places. *Journal of Philosophy of Education*, 34(1), 183–96.

Boynton, P., Swinglehurst, D., Greenhalgh, T. *et al.* (2005) Our course and winning the THES/Academy eTutor award 2005. Available from: www.medev.ac.uk/newsletter/article/126/ (accessed 9 April 2012).

Brown, A. and Dowling, P. (1998) *Doing Research/Reading Research: a mode of interrogation for education*. London, Falmer Press.

Bruner, J. (1985) Narrative and paradigmatic modes of thought. In: E. Eisner (ed.) *Learning and Teaching the Ways of Knowing*. Chicago, IL, University of Chicago Press, pp.97–115.

Clandinin, D. and Connelly, F. (2000) *Narrative Inquiry*. San Francisco, CA, Jossey-Bass.

Conole, G., de Laat, M., Dillon, T., *et al.* (2008) 'Disruptive technologies', 'pedagogical innovation': what's new? Findings from an in-depth study of students use and perceptions of technology. *Computers and Education*, 50(2), 511–24.

Cortazzi, M. (2001) Narrative learning in clinical and other contexts. Presented at the Brunel University Education Department Research Conference, London, UK 17–18 July.

Creanor, L., Trinder, K., Gowan, D. *et al.* (2006) *LEX: the learner experience of e-learning: final project report*. Available from: www.jisc.ac.uk/uploaded_documents/LEX%20Final%20Report_August06.pdf (accessed 9 April 2012).

Czarniawska, B. (2004) *Narratives in Social Science Research*. London, Sage.

Daly, C., Pachler, N., Pickering, J., *et al.* (2007) Teachers as e-learners: exploring the experiences of teachers in an online professional master's programme. *Journal of In-Service Education*, 33(4), 443–61.

Decortis, F. (2004) *Survey of Narrative Theories for Learning Environments*. Brussels, European Commission, Kaleidoscope. Available from: http://telearn.noe-kaleidoscope.org/warehouse/Decortis-Kaleidoscope-2005.pdf (accessed 9 April 2012).

Eagleton, T. (2003) *After Theory*. London, Penguin Allen Lane.

Elliott, J. (2005) *Using Narrative in Social Research: qualitative and quantitative approaches*. London, Sage.

Greenhalgh, T. (2006) *What Seems to Be the Trouble? Stories in illness and healthcare*. Oxford, Radcliffe Publishing.

Greenhalgh, T. and Hurwitz, B. (1999) Narrative based medicine: why study narrative? *British Medical Journal*, 318(7175), 48–50.

Greenhalgh, T., Russell, J. and Swinglehurst, D. (2005) Narrative methods in quality improvement research. *Quality and Safety in Health Care*, 14(6), 443–9.

Gubrium, J. (2003) *Postmodern Interviewing*. London, Sage.

Hall, R. (2008) Digital inclusion: evaluation. Presentation at Futurelab Research Discussion Day, London, UK 20 March.

Levy, P. (2006) "Living" theory: a pedagogical framework for process support in networked learning. *ALT J, Research in Learning Technology*, 14(3), 225–40.

Luckin, R., Plowman, L., Laurillard, D., *et al.* (2001) Narrative evolution: learning from students' talk about species variation. *International Journal of Artificial Intelligence in Education*, 12(1), 100–123. Available from: http://eprints.ioe.ac.uk/205/1/Luckin2001Narrative100.pdf (accessed 9 April 2012).

Lyotard, F. (1984) *The Postmodern Condition: a report on knowledge*. Manchester, Manchester University Press.

McConnell, D. (2006) *E-Learning Groups and Communities*. Maidenhead, Open University Press.

McCracken, G. (1988) *The Long Interview*. Newbury Park, Sage.

Polkinghorne, D. (1988) *Narrative Knowing and the Human Sciences*. New York, NY, State University of New York Press.

Prosser, M. (2005) Why we shouldn't use student surveys of teaching as satisfaction ratings. Available from: www.heacademy.ac.uk/resources/detail/subjects/bioscience/nss-satisfaction-ratings (accessed 9 April 2012).

Richardson, J. T. E. (2005) Instruments for obtaining student feedback: a review of the literature. *Assessment and Evaluation in Higher Education*, 30(4), 387–415.

Sharpe, R., Benfield, G., Lessner, E. *et al.* (2005) Scoping study for the pedagogy strand of the JISC e-learning programme. Available from: www.jisc.ac.uk/uploaded_documents/scoping%20study%20final%20report%20v4.1.doc (accessed 9 April 2012).

Sharples, M. (2007) An interactional model of context. Presentation at the Philosophy of Technology-Enhanced Learning seminar, 29 June, London Knowledge Lab.

11

Review

Communication, knowing and being in work-based learning

Tim Dornan

Introduction

The previous 10 chapters have shown how work-based learning theory can help researchers frame their investigations into the education of health professionals. The research reported in these chapters was conducted in a range of educational practices: medical students' learning in firms (Chapter 1), medical educators' learning on the job (Chapter 2), nursing education and practice (Chapters 4 and 6), the development of clinical teachers (Chapter 5), learning in operating theatres (Chapter 7), optometry practice (Chapter 9), and online study in a professional masters programme (Chapter 10). One (Chapter 8) explains how actor-network theory can be used to investigate whole multi-professional systems of practice. Another (Chapter 3) provides an important counterpoint to all the other chapters by taking work-based assessment as a main focus and exploring its relationship with practice-based learning. The main theoretical perspectives of the book are communities of practice (Chapter 1), Eraut's and Billett's work-based learning frameworks (Chapters 2 and 3, respectively), Bernstein's sociology of education (Chapter 4), activity theory (Chapter 5), social semiotics (Chapter 7), actor-network theory (Chapter 8), ethnomethodology (Chapter 9), and narrative research (Chapter 10). Chapter 6 argues for using multiple theoretical perspectives. This final chapter is a synthesis that cuts across the topics of all the earlier chapters. It presents them as instances of two unitary perspectives on work-based learning, which I term 'process within context' and 'ways of knowing'. Whereas both perspectives are primarily focused on learning processes, Chapter 3's focus on workplace assessment also emphasises the 'products' of learning in the form of standardised competencies. This review chapter is not so concerned with research methodologies as with the pedagogy of work-based learning, so it leaves the 10 excellent descriptions of how authors arrived at their insights to speak for themselves. The editors' intention was that this book would close the gap between abstract socio-cultural theory and its application to the problems of health professionals' education so the chapter ends by suggesting some implications for practice.

Process within context

Vignettes

This section presents five of the chapters that clearly illustrate the theme of 'process within context', synthesised in the form of *vignettes*. These are constructed around core constitutive elements found in each of the chapters: theoretical orientation, the unit of analysis, process, learning, context and results.

Chapter 1 has a theoretical orientation toward communities of practice theory, and its unit of analysis is, unsurprisingly, a community of people engaged in practice. The central process is participation in shared, social practice. Learning is an integral and inseparable part *of* practice; learners are 'legitimate peripheral participants' *in* practice. The context has physical and cultural features; so, for example, outpatient departments, wards, and operating theatres are places in which culturally determined events like clinics, ward rounds and surgical operations take place. The result of participation in practice within those contexts is for learners to construct identities. An important feature of learning, from a communities of practice perspective, is that identity does not just develop as a result of but *is* membership of a community, and ability to demonstrate certain skills, which afford further participation. So, identity is a social process more than a commodity acquired by learners.

Chapter 2 has a theoretical orientation toward Eraut's framework of practice-based learning. Its unit of analysis is an individual person learning through work. The process is individual action within a social context, such as completing tasks and observing practice. Learning is integral to individual and collective action; it involves whole people and is fostered by reflection on what they experienced and how they reacted, emotionally, to those experiences. The context is activity within workplaces, which vary in how conducive they are to learning. One result of workplace learning is to recognise and manage emotions; others are to understand and be able to respond sensitively to other people and 'perform' (in an artistic sense) a craft. An important feature of learning, from Eraut's perspective, is how learners progress along 'trajectories' of expert performance.

Chapter 5 has a theoretical orientation toward activity theory, and takes, as its unit of analysis, an activity system that may be on an even larger scale than a single community. The process of interest is activity, defined as a collection of subjects conjointly directing their will toward an object. Learning results from participation in the activity, but it defies general description beyond that. The context of the activity is a community with its own cultural history, division of labour, tools and rules. An important feature of activity systems is the capacity for several of them to exist within a single social context and for contradictions to exist between them, resolution of which opens up potential for expansive transformations in learning.

Chapter 7 has a theoretical orientation toward social semiotics. Its unit of analysis is people with individual identities and social roles who are engaged as co-actors in social practices. The central process is interaction between people, focusing particularly on the processes of communication that make up those interactions. Learning is located within communication practices as well as within the minds of those who communicate. It is described as 'principled engagement with a multimodal environment'. Actors learn to use a variety of different modes of communication appropriately in different situations. Contexts within which they do so are the many different sites in which medicine is practised: wards, operating theatres, trauma bays and so on. An important feature of those places is their social organisation: who the participants are, their relations, what power is at issue, what social purposes have been assigned to the sites, and in what ways those purposes are exercised. The results of interaction are adopting social roles and performing communicative acts by means of speech, body postures, touch and so on. Changes take place in actors' understandings of their social worlds and the way they interpret communicative acts, which demonstrate what they have yet to learn. An important feature of learning, from a social semiotic perspective, is that social actors shape learning environments in such a way that context, process and outcome are inseparably linked in a dynamic relationship.

Chapter 8 has a theoretical orientation toward actor-network theory. Its unit of analysis is a network – a social system, which can be of any size. The central processes are formation, widening and strengthening of networks. Learning is integral to network formation since networks are purposefully fostered to produce knowledge and transform practice. Context, which has a prominent place in the theory, includes physical artefacts as well as human 'actors in the drama of learning'. The results of network formation can include (social) climate change. An important feature of actor-network theory is that a most important 'result' is the network itself, which creates alliances and has translation effects across an unpredictable number of persons, material objects and ideas. Work-nets of this sort leave traces behind, which can be viewed as their 'results'.

Synthesis

The preceding vignettes are not essentially different from one another, because any single workplace could be viewed from any or all of the five perspectives. The five different theoretical orientations can be thought of as the different powered lenses of a socio-cultural microscope, which is being used to examine learning processes. Activity theory, the lowest-power lens, gives the broadest field of analysis, while social semiotics is the highest power, and gives the most detailed focus. The learning processes that can be seen through the various lenses are all participatory, bringing together people with different levels of expertise in activities that 'get the job done' and from which all parties learn. The five different processes all make learning inseparable from practice, although there is one important qualitative difference between them. Eraut's framework of practice-based learning, social semiotics and (as discussed in the next section) Billett's framework are theories of mind as well as of social practice, whereas the other theories locate learning more or less solely within social practice. From all perspectives, communicative practices have an important part in learning processes. Contexts have social and material features that do not just interact with but *constitute* learning processes. The result of those processes (I deliberately avoid the word 'outcome', for reasons explained in the next section) is formation of professional identity, which includes the ability to engage in practice, learn from it and develop as an individual. The five perspectives all represent learning as a dynamic, non-standard, contextualised process, which changes people's ways of being in the world.

'Outcomes' and assessment

References to assessment are more or less confined to Chapter 3, which provides a much-needed counterpoint to the other chapters by exploring how assessment and learning processes relate to each other. Since the chapter stands alone in setting out to reconcile assessment with workplace learning theory, and the relationship between the two is of considerable interest, this commentary first presents the chapter contents in the same synthetic way as for the other chapters and then traces the discourse of assessment within it.

Chapter 3 has a theoretical orientation toward Billett's framework of practice-based learning, drawing also on Piaget's cognitive learning theory. The unit of analysis is individual learners who act as 'agents' in pursuit of workplace learning opportunities and construct knowledge consequent on their workplace experiences. The central process is conducting work tasks under close supervision and guidance from colleagues and experts. Learning has both a behavioural component – seeking out and engaging with opportunities – and a cognitive component – the products of everyday thinking and acting. People develop their cognitive structures by making sense of situations they encounter during work. The context is workplaces, which vary in their social structures, division of labour and lines of accountability, and influence learning for better or worse. The result is that learners develop expertise and move from simple tasks with low accountability to more complex tasks with higher accountability. An important feature of Billett's framework is guidance by experts in learning at work. This occurs at three levels: the first is organising and managing learners' experiences in workplaces; the second is modelling key tasks and demonstrating procedures; the third is developing self-regulated learning and transferring knowledge and skills to other workplaces.

Chapter 3 equates Billett's first level of 'creating a curriculum and opportunities at the workplace for learners to perform the tasks required for them to progress within the profession' with 'identifying core competencies that should be acquired at progressive stages of training'. Since regulatory bodies such as the one that commissioned the research in Chapter 3 have dictated that doctors cannot progress within the profession unless they demonstrate such competencies, nobody can disagree with that equation, but just how strong are the arguments for using core competencies to organise and manage learners' experiences in workplaces? It is argued elsewhere (Mørcke et al., in preparation) that the notion of core competencies arose from a regulatory discourse of professional education and there is a lack of well-theorised practical evidence that links it with teaching and learning activities. The anecdote in Chapter 1 of the consultant who asked a learner if he was measuring blood pressure as if for the objective structured clinical examination (OSCE) or as a doctor would measure it, graphically illustrates the tension between real practice and competencies standardised for assessment purposes. The chapter goes on to equate Billett's second level of 'guidance in the development of procedures' and his third level of 'developing self-regulated learning and ability to transfer knowledge and skills to other workplaces' with formative assessment. The analysis concludes that there are important parallels between Billett's framework and assessment regimes for specialty training, but notes the difficulty of ensuring that suitably qualified experts are available at the point of delivery of clinical care to provide appropriate guidance and formative feedback. It acknowledges that the relationship between assessment and learning may be tilted unduly toward assessment. It reports findings from empirical research that the process may be subverted by learners choosing 'doves' rather than 'hawks' to assess them, that supervisors are reluctant to offer formative assessment of routine procedures, and that the process can indeed become trivialised to a tick-box activity.

This analysis begs the question whether assessing the product of learning, in the form of core competencies, can truly help learners progress within the profession in the most complex sense of becoming experts. Chapter 5 reminds us of Sfard's distinction between the 'learning-as-acquisition' and 'learning-as-participation' metaphors and quotes Bleakley's argument that there is a productive tension between these competing ideas that requires us to choose the educational perspective that has the most explanatory power for issues being explored. It then pursues an accommodation between the participation (process) and acquisition (product) metaphors by exploring the second main argument of this chapter, that work-based learning concerns a rich variety of 'ways of knowing'. If we understood them better, perhaps we could populate our curricula with more valid and acceptable acquisitions than competencies that seem, according to Chapter 3, to be treated with equal disdain by supervisors and learners.

Ways of knowing

Vignettes

The four chapters I have not yet discussed exemplify different ways of knowing.

Chapter 4 has a theoretical orientation toward Bernstein's sociology of education; its context is the practice of UK nurse education. The medium of nurses' knowing, according to this analysis, is participation in work-based curricula. Nursing is, according to Bernstein's classification, a 'weakly classified field'; in other words, there is great uncertainty about what 'official curricula' should contain and how they should be structured. As a result, there is heavy reliance on learning requirements handed down by professional bodies. Chapter 4 identifies three distinct ways of knowing in the nursing domain: (1) the propositional discourses and knowledge structures produced by the small number of people who 'use the distribution rules of the field to frame a canon of literature and reify some discourses over others to create dominant, higher-status' knowledge bases; (2) teachers must 'recontextualise' the prescribed knowledge base into a format that makes it possible for learners to demonstrate attainment of 'demonstrable learning outcomes that … are reliable, valid and transferable to … the practice domain'; (3) the 'profane or practice-based knowledges of those engaged in the field of reproduction (practice)'. Chapter 4 refers repeatedly to a tension between profane and arcane ways of knowing, highlighting that practitioners 'need to draw upon a repertoire of knowledge, the relevance of which may not have been apparent at the time of its acquisition'. There is also a tension between ways of knowing learnt in different environments, the result being that nurses develop highly situated and context-dependent sets of case exemplars. They reproduce 'social relations, forms of consciousness, role identity and professional habitus rather than reified knowledge structures; that is, what it "means" to be a nurse and how a nurse should "behave", rather than what they should "know"'.

While Chapter 6 has an eclectic theoretical orientation, its conceptualisation of ways of knowing draws particularly on the work of Polanyi and Rorty. Its context is nursing practice with a focus on tacit knowledge, in which 'the personal participation of the knower is essential in all acts of understanding. Knowing is a skilful action requiring an active comprehension of the known.' Polanyi recognised 'focal' and 'subsidiary' kinds of knowing, attention being focused on the focal while the subsidiary is part of a person's general awareness. He writes of an art of knowing which can be communicated only by example. Rorty defined intuition as 'immediate apprehension', which includes sensation, knowledge and mystical rapport. He noted distinct differences among the following terms: hunches – 'unjustified true belief not preceded by inference'; 'immediate knowledge of the truth' – knowledge not preceded by inference and not related to knowledge of a concept; and 'immediate knowledge of a concept' – occasions when knowledge is not accompanied by an ability to define it. Finally, he referred to 'nonpropositional' knowledge of an entity where, although knowledge is a necessary condition for the intuition of the entity, it may be sense perceptions, intuitions about universals and mystical or inexpressible intuitions. All in all, Chapter 6 identifies a facet of professional knowing that is tacit and embodied and for which active participation and active integration of new with previous experience are requisite. It distinguishes 'mere competence' from expertise acquired through participation in practice, under the tutelage of an experienced practitioner. There is an affective dimension to tacit knowledge, in that concepts like 'hope', 'commitment', 'obligation' and 'responsibility' are associated with personal knowing. Chapter 6 regards learning in healthcare workplaces as concerned with learning in action for action; learners need to develop skills of imagination and improvisation, and they need to be open to new possibilities that can arise from the adoption, adaptation or reconstruction of existing theory, tools and practices.

Chapter 9 has a theoretical orientation toward workplace studies and ethnomethodology. Its context is optometry practice. It describes how common-sense knowledge about everyday events is embedded in work activities. This type of knowledge includes contextual details of real-world actions and practical knowledge of the ways people go about accomplishing tasks. It includes, also, knowledge of the resources people use to do their work and the social organisation of particular contexts. Common-sense knowledge is a largely tacit, taken-for-granted and intuitively known feature of action. It is not easily articulated verbally and can only be gained by undertaking the activity to which it pertains, rather than by studying in the abstract. Communication skills have an important place in professional knowing, since optometric consultations are co-produced through the interaction between optometrists and patients. An important part of learning to become a clinician involves not only learning technical, clinical knowledge but also learning to apply and use that knowledge in practice. A good deal of the competencies required for a given area of professional practice are learnt through engaging in the work itself.

Chapter 10 has a theoretical orientation towards narrative research. Its context is online learning discussion groups in an international primary healthcare masters programme. Participants are busy practitioners from different health professions, different countries and different work settings, often isolated from other health professionals, and only meeting one another online. They are undertaking professional learning alongside their work roles. They take ownership of their learning processes, controlling the timing and location of their engagement and presenting online 'personas'. The medium of their knowing is narrative, which they contribute to a collective process of building knowledge and learning. This way of knowing is described as 'experiencing experience'. Narrative is a medium that allows participants' learning to remain deeply rooted in the contexts in which events took place. It allows them consciously to examine their workplace experiences from different perspectives, interpreting what they see creatively, drawing on their tacit understanding; they capture, articulate, reconstruct and project remembered experience. They organise it into temporarily meaningful episodes, telling stories to explain their actions and those of others. By doing so, narrative becomes a medium to explore complex human experience, making sense and meaning from it. By imposing an interpretive framework, narrative allows participants to communicate and share experiences, views and interpretations. With the help of other learners, narrative is a medium for them to deepen their self-awareness, critically review their professional selves, construct professional knowledge and transform their professional identities, including knowledge and skills. In contrast to 'logico-scientific and empirical truth', narrative is a medium that can accommodate multiple versions of reality, challenging 'common sense' versions of professional identity and practice.

Synthesis

There is remarkable consistency between the four chapters that 'knowing' in work-based health professionals' education is at least as much a process as a product. Knowing is a skilful and creative process of interpreting new experiences, integrating them with pre-existing tacit knowledge, organising, constructing and projecting understanding. Knowing involves communicating with peer learners, tutors and patients. People tell stories to explain their actions and use narrative as a medium to explore and make sense of their experiences. By communicating their knowing, learners deepen their self-awareness, critically review their professional selves, construct their knowledge and transform their identities. Viewed as *product* rather than process, professional knowing is profane rather than arcane. Work-based knowing is contextualised to practice settings and embedded in practices. It is oral, local and multilayered. It includes common sense and uncommon sense. It exists as scripts. It includes knowing how people go about real-world tasks, the resources they draw on to do so, and the way practice contexts are organised. In contrast to scientific knowledge, professional knowing can accommodate multiple versions of reality and professional identities that are as many and varied as the people who have them. The product of work-based learning is tacit as well as declarative. It includes hunch, non-propositional knowledge and taken-for-granted features of action. It has an affective as well as a cognitive dimension. It is not fundamentally at odds with the formal knowledge of 'school', but it contextualises and applies that type of knowledge to practice. Work-based learning may, in addition, free people from formal knowledge. Through their work-based experience, learners discover new ways of acting, social relations, forms of consciousness and role identities: what it means to be a health professional and how one should behave rather than what one should know. People develop ways of knowing through example more than by precept. They learn action though action, improvise, adapt and reconstruct what they observe. Work plays a central part in professional learning because it is only by undertaking an activity that it can be learnt.

Implications

This section draws together strands teased out earlier in this chapter to identify some practical implications. The first part of this chapter proposed that work-based learning is a dynamic, non-standard, contextualised process that changes people's ways of being in the world. The second part proposed that work-based learning entails many different ways of knowing. From a socio-cultural perspective, 'ways of being' and 'ways of knowing' are not far removed from one another and become one in the communicative practices of workgroups, which have such a prominent place in this book. But two problems remain. The first was identified in Chapter 1, which reminded us that Sfard identified two dominant metaphors for learning and argued that 'too great a devotion to one particular metaphor can lead to theoretical distortions and to undesirable practices' (Sfard, 1998, p.4). This book is devoted to Sfard's 'participation metaphor' more than her 'acquisition metaphor', and even when the latter was introduced in Chapter 3 in the treatment of core competencies, I have suggested that this is problematic. The second problem, which is the main topic of Chapter 3, is how to assess work-based learning in a valid way. Those two related problems might be characterised in Sfard's words as a refusal by the authors of this book, with a few exceptions, to 'reify knowledge'. The counterargument, I suggest, is to be found Chapter 4, which distinguishes the arcane knowledge of curricula from the profane knowledge of workplaces and describes the contortions educators have to go through to link the two. The profane professional knowledge described in this book is so complex that it would pose a formidable challenge to any typologist determined to reify it. Even if the typologist were successful, there is an additional problem. Learning never reaches a clearly definable endpoint, but proceeds dynamically along a lifelong learning continuum. That may be why both teachers and learners treat competency frameworks, as currently formulated, with such disdain.

But assessment and accountability will not go away and nor should they. Rather than reject attempts to codify professional knowledge as futile, it is the social responsibility of professionals to continue exploring it. Within the field of mathematics education, Williams has distinguished the 'use value' of mathematics from its 'exchange value' (Williams, 2011). The anecdote of the consultant and measurement of blood pressure illustrates the concept well. Measuring blood pressure like a doctor has 'use value' because it can be used to care for patients; measuring it for the OSCE has 'exchange value', because demonstrating the ability to do it can be exchanged for a diploma, which confers the right to practise as a doctor. In an ideal educational world, use and exchange values would not be so far removed from one another. The world as it now exists, the OSCE anecdote suggests, is not yet ideal.

The 10 research case studies presented here illustrate very clearly how learning theory can inform research methodology, and they provide a rich resource for researchers to draw on in framing and theorising their research topics and choosing appropriate methodologies. My argument leads me to conclude that assessment of workplace proficiency is a burning issue in workplace learning research, particularly as regards (re)licensure of physicians. Until recently, licensure depended on learners completing prescribed periods of training and passing tests that had dubious validity and reliability. Completion of training is no longer regarded as sufficient evidence for licensure, and competence must be demonstrated in reliable tests. But, given the complex relationship between process, context and different ways of knowing, what do we mean by competence? There, I suggest, is an important research agenda.

Finally, what are the implications for practice? Reassuringly, the case studies present a strong argument for maintaining the status quo. Practice is learnt in and through practice. The authors have reinforced the importance of that truth by showing some of the ways in which work-based experience can be educational. The purpose of critical scholarship, however, should not so much be to maintain the status quo as to identify ways of improving it. If I were to choose one message from this book that could strengthen educational practice it is the observation that learning is embedded in the communicative practices of workgroups. The contributors have identified many different uses of the spoken word and other forms of communication that contribute to learning. Let us attend to how our ways of being and knowing are present in our communication with one another and explore how we can identify, strengthen and share the essence of good clinical practice.

References

Mørcke, A. M., Eika B. and Dornan, T. (in preparation) Critical review of how an outcome-based approach affects undergraduate medical teaching and learning [provisional title]. Draft copy available from the author of this chapter.

Sfard, A. (1998) On two metaphors for learning and the dangers of choosing just one. *Educational Researcher*, 27(2), 4–13.

Williams, J. (2011) Use and exchange value in mathematics education: contemporary CHAT meets Bourdieu's sociology. *Educational Studies in Mathematics*, 80(1–2), 57–72.

Index

Entries in **bold** refer to figures and tables.

Index

Index

Index

talk
  learning to 14–15, 19
  organisation of 168
teachers
  authority of 129
  engagement with education 30
  evaluation of 77
  and recontextualisation 67
teaching
  as activity system **89**
  constitution of community 94
  emotional challenge in 37
  logic of 74
  as mediated activity **88**
  as social practice 125
  spoken commentary as 136
  suboptimal 38
  technocratic organisation of 94
  and work activity 33
teaching practices, *see* pedagogical practices
teaching skills 85
teams, in ANT 148
teamwork, improving 151
technology
  deploying 172
  and lifelong learning 190
tensions, creative 97
texts, interpreting 116, 196
think aloud techniques 112–13
thinking
  higher-order 70
  and knowing 111
  in social practice 13–14
thinking-in-action 104, 110, 112
TIRA (tacit, intuition and reflection/knowing-in-action) 105, 120
tokens 148
Tomorrow's Doctors 11, 92–4
trades unions 7
trainee doctors
  assessment of 50–1, 54–60
  coaching of 49–50
  curriculum for 49
  learning to talk 20
  'practising' on patients 87
  reflection by 59
  responsibility of 47, 51–2
  supervision of 45
  and surgery 133

training, and practice 169–70
transcription systems 172–4, **176**
transformation, expansive 87, 91, 97, 209
translations
  in ANT 146, 148–9
  visibility of 159
transmitter–acquirer relationship 67
truth, and narrative 192–4
TTRM (Theatre Team Resource Management) 151–4, 159–62

unknowing, patterns of 113
user reference groups 6

venepuncture 14
verisimilitude 192, 203
video recordings, in workplace studies 172–3, 184
visual problems, description of 174, **175**, 179, 182–3
Vygotsky, Lev 88

wakefulness, maintaining 200
ward round teaching **88–9**
ways of being 216
ways of knowing
  and epistemology 115
  and narrative 192
  and WBL 208, 212
  and work organisations 5
web designers 160
websites 149, 151, 157, 160
Wenger, Etienne 12
Wikipedia 164
wisdom, practical 112, 145
work activities, *see* work practices
work-based learning (WBL)
  activities of 30
  and ANT 149
  approaches to study of 29
  content of 30–1
  and creative technologies 9
  desirability of 41
  different conceptions of 3
  formal and informal 28–9, 36
  as mature field 1–2
  in medical settings 33–4, 39
  multi-dimensional influences on 40

opportunities for 38–9, 41
tacit 34
and transferability of skills 72
triggering of 5–6, 29
unitary perspectives on 207–8
and ways of knowing 216
work contexts, purposes derived from **7**
work experience 3, 197
work–learning relationship 2–3
work-nets
  and networks 149
  retracing of 150
  strengthening 154
work practices
  habitual 152
  learning from 29–30, 32, 39, 100
  routine and non-routine 46–8
  and tacit knowledge 171
  in workplace studies 169
workplace assessment
  in medicine 53–8, 61
  processes of 45, 50–1, 56
  products of 208
  reflection in 58–9
  tools for 59–60
workplace learning
  and assessment 45
  Billet's model of 46–50, 53
  and expertise 46
  organisation of 183
  for teachers 38
  and TIRA 120
  trajectories of **31**, 32, 35–6, **37**, 39–41
  and WBL 3–4
workplace rules 5
workplace studies
  definition of 167–8
  detail in 170
  and medicine 169
  methodology of 172–3
  and tacit knowledge 171, 183–4
workplaces
  conversation in 30
  cultures of 7, 41
  learning opportunities in 32–3
  micro-interactions in 4